More Praise for *The A₁ Homeopathy Handb*

D0770587

"Children will thank parents and pediatric̶ ̶ ̶ ̶ ̶ ̶ book and use homeopathy as a safe and valuable method to treat their acute and chronic health problems. More important, Dr. Shalts informs parents that children with acute health problems who are treated and healed with homeopathy are more resilient and therefore less likely to develop a chronic illness."

—Lawrence B. Palevsky, M.D., F.A.A.P., president, American Holistic Medical Association

"Dr. Shalts accomplishes a great deal in one book. He presents a history of homeopathy, explains what to expect in a homeopathic interview, and delves into home treatment. The case descriptions are compelling and create a feeling as though Dr. Shalts is speaking to each parent individually. Great job!"

—Amy Rothenberg, N.D., D.H.A.N.P., and Paul Herscu, N.D., D.H.A.N.P., cofounders and principal instructors, New England School of Homeopathy

"Dr. Shalts's *Handbook* has made homeopathy more accessible with its clear and concise description of the practical uses of this potent medical therapy. Effective for all ages and a wide range of illnesses, homeopathy can now be part of every family's home first-aid kit and part of every patient's choice for treatment of many common conditions with this book's recommendations."

—Robert Schiller, M.D., chairman, Department of Family Medicine, Beth Israel Medical Center; assistant professor, department of family medicine, Albert Einstein College of Medicine; senior vice president, Institute for Urban Family Health

"Edward Shalts is one of the nation's most gifted homeopathic physicians. As an M.D. trained in both family medicine and psychiatry, he has written the definitive family guide to homeopathy, suitable for practitioners, consumers, and especially parents. This is a must-have reference guide in homeopathy."

—Woodson C. Merrell, M.D., M. Anthony Fisher Director of Integrative Medicine, Continuum Center for Health and Healing, Beth Israel Medical Center; assistant clinical professor of medicine, Columbia University, College of Physicians and Surgeons

The American Institute of Homeopathy Handbook for Parents

The American Institute of Homeopathy Handbook for Parents

A Guide to Healthy Treatment for Everything from Colds and Allergies to ADHD, Obesity, and Depression

Edward Shalts, M.D., D.Ht.

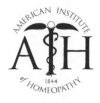

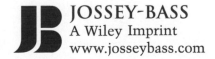

JOSSEY-BASS
A Wiley Imprint
www.josseybass.com

Published by Jossey-Bass
A Wiley Imprint
989 Market Street, San Francisco, CA 94103-1741   www.josseybass.com

The contents of this work are intended to further general scientific research, understanding, and discussion only and are not intended and should not be relied upon as recommending or promoting a specific method, diagnosis, or treatment by physicians for any particular patient. The publisher and the author make no representations or warranties with respect to the accuracy or completeness of the contents of this work and specifically disclaim all warranties, including without limitation any implied warranties of fitness for a particular purpose. In view of ongoing research, equipment modifications, changes in governmental regulations, and the constant flow of information relating to the use of medicines, equipment, and devices, the reader is urged to review and evaluate the information provided in the package insert or instructions for each medicine, equipment, or device for, among other things, any changes in the instructions or indication of usage and for added warnings and precautions. Readers should consult with a specialist where appropriate. All case studies herein are based on composites of real case studies and are intended to provide general information, rather than to represent real individuals or specific situations. The fact that an organization or Web site is referred to in this work as a citation and/or a potential source of further information does not mean that the author or the publisher endorses the information the organization or Web site may provide or recommendations it may make. Further, readers should be aware that Internet Web sites listed in this work may have changed or disappeared between when this work was written and when it is read. No warranty may be created or extended by any promotional statements for this work. Neither the publisher nor the author shall be liable for any damages arising herefrom.

Jossey-Bass books and products are available through most bookstores. To contact Jossey-Bass directly, call our Customer Care Department within the U.S. at 800-956-7739, outside the U.S. at 317-572-3986, or fax 317-572-4002.

Jossey-Bass also publishes its books in a variety of electronic formats. Some content that appears in print may not be available in electronic books.

Library of Congress Cataloging-in-Publication Data
Shalts, Edward, date.
  The American Institute of Homeopathy handbook for parents : a guide to healthy treatment for everything from colds and allergies to ADHD, obesity, and depression / Edward Shalts.
    p. cm.
  Includes bibliographical references and index.
  ISBN-13 978-0-7879-8033-7 (alk. paper)
  ISBN-10 0-7879-8033-1 (alk. paper)
  1. Children—Diseases—Homeopathic treatment—Popular works. 2. Homeopathy—Popular works. I. American Institute of Homeopathy. II. Title.
  RX503.S53 2005
  615.5'32'083—dc22
                              2005014315

Printed in the United States of America
FIRST EDITION
PB Printing   10 9 8 7 6 5 4 3 2 1

Contents

To my beloved daughters, Dora and Polina

Acknowledgments

First, I am grateful to Alan Rinzler at Jossey-Bass, who came up with the idea for this book and together with Catherine Craddock continually encouraged and supported the high quality of the editorial work. I would also like to thank production editor Carol Hartland, copyeditor Marcy Marsh, and marketing manager Jennifer Wenzel.

I am grateful to the board of trustees of the American Institute of Homeopathy for providing me with the opportunity to write this handbook on behalf of the organization. My sincere gratitude also extends to Rona Lichtenberg, who opened my eyes to the possibility of writing and encouraged me to take my first steps in this direction. The other person who constantly dreamed about my writing a book was my late father, Boris. I hope there is a way for him to celebrate this book with all of us, wherever he is at the moment.

Writing this book would not have been possible without the encouragement, nurture, and unconditional love that I constantly receive from my dear wife, Natasha. I also want to thank my daughters, Dora and Polina, for keeping the volume of our TV as low as they could during the writing process, and just for being there for me to love and admire. I appreciate all of the carbohydrates and other support provided by my mother, Emma.

I have the highest regard for the extraordinary writing, editorial, and organizational skills of Stephanie Gunning. Without her brilliant work, this book would not speak to readers in such an inviting and easy-to-comprehend language.

I truly appreciate the efforts and exceptional communication skills provided by Stephany Evans, my literary agent.

I am very grateful to Dr. Joyce Frye, Dr. Paul Herscu, and Dr. George Guess for reviewing this book and providing valuable suggestions. Special acknowledgment is also due to Paul Herscu and George Vithoulkas for providing me with important insights on the core issues of homeopathy.

I would like to thank Mr. Sow for all his support and Dr. Amy Rothenberg for helping me always to think about horses, not zebras, each time I hear hooves. Thanks also to Julian Winston for writing and publishing his great book, *The Faces of Homeopathy*, which made searching for information on the history of homeopathy so easy and a lot of fun.

The American Institute of Homeopathy Handbook for Parents

Introduction

What Can Homeopathy Do for Your Children?

The American Institute of Homeopathy Handbook for Parents is designed to offer you a healthy alternative to conventional medical treatments for your children's ailments.

Homeopathy is a medical specialty that uses natural substances, known as *remedies*, which are diluted and shaken in order to stimulate the body's natural healing abilities. According to the principle of *similars* (discussed in Chapter One), which is the foundation of this approach, a substance that causes a combination of symptoms in a healthy, sensitive individual will cure similar symptoms in the sick. Homeopathy has been proven effective in the treatment of acute ailments, such as colic, fevers, and ear infections, as well as in the treatment of chronic diseases, such as asthma, depression, and allergies. Practitioners interview patients, usually for a few hours, in order to pinpoint the exact remedy that's needed. Homeopathy completely sidesteps the potential harms of more radical interventions.

Unlike conventional drugs, homeopathic remedies have a two hundred–year record of being able to provide individualized help and highly effective cures for many illnesses without causing any side effects or complications. They are also easy to use.

The Current Crisis

Numerous health experts in the United States and around the world warn that within a generation—if left unchecked—a worrying trend of parents looking after sick children could increase even beyond its current alarming level. These days, in addition to traditional childhood diseases, our sons and daughters are being diagnosed too frequently with a variety of physical and mental health problems that include allergies, asthma, obesity, sinusitis, ear infections, attention deficit–hyperactivity disorder (ADHD), autism, and depression.

According to a report issued by the U.S. Surgeon General's Office in 2000, the burden of suffering experienced by sick children and their families has created a major crisis. For despite widespread acknowledgment of these problems and many extreme efforts to treat them, children's illnesses are still on the rise. Whatever we're doing collectively to overcome this public health emergency is, frankly, not working.

Like a giant with legs made of clay, powerful conventional medications have failed to provide a universal answer to the growing epidemic of emotional and physical problems that our children are experiencing. Prozac and Ritalin have become cultural icons, illustrating both our desire to medicate children for expediency and the failure of our search for miracle drugs. Instead of being tools of last resort, many potent psychotropics, hormones, and antibiotics are used unreasonably often, and this has led to numerous side effects and unnecessary complications. In fact, drugs are now one of the most significant factors in an overall environmental assault on children's health that's under way in our culture. Furthermore, because of the tremendous promise that doctors and parents hoped and believed these medications offered us, tremendous disappointment ensued when the anticipated miracle did not happen.

Fortunately, there is another, better option for parents, such as you, who have recognized the wisdom of resisting the overuse of drugs like antibiotics, steroids, and psychotropic medications in treating childhood diseases. Homeopathy is that option.

The Homeopathic Solution

Homeopathy not only cures diseases, but it does so by boosting the functions of the body's major integrative systems. Every time children overcome acute ailments with only a little help from a homeopathic remedy, their defense mechanisms are strengthened. Soon their immune systems are able to fight off infections without any help at all. They become free of illness and independent of medications. Reliance on conventional drugs, by contrast, weakens children's major defense mechanisms and leads to their increased dependence on drugs and other interventions. A vicious cycle results, as one illness and its treatment lead inexorably to another, and health problems become more systemic.

Homeopathy is extremely safe, because it is a hit-or-miss proposition. Remedies must be given with a high degree of precision or else they won't work or produce any effects at all. Conventional medicine cannot offer this level of precision. Not even close! In contrast with targeting only what is wrong in the body, drugs attack both illness and host, causing an enormous amount of collateral damage. The numerous side effects of steroids, antibiotics, and even over-the-counter medications for the common cold are not a secret. Everybody knows about them. Recent studies indicate that one of the significant side effects of antidepressants is increased suicidal behavior. For caring and responsible parents, these sorts of adverse consequences for their children are worrisome and unacceptable.

The problems of side effects don't necessarily stop after taking one medication. Secondary medications are often required to counteract the side effects caused by an originally prescribed drug. These drugs have their own side effects, so problems continue to pile up. It is a bad enough outcome in adult medicine. For children, the situation is worse. Children are growing and their bodies have significantly more plasticity. Negative effects from various interventions make a long-lasting impact on their development.

Children come without manuals. Fortunately, homeopathy provides a blueprint for how things work in the human body and what to do in case things begin to break.

The main point of this handbook is to explain homeopathy's unique perspective on issues of health and disease, an approach that will enable you to understand your children's true state of health better. Armed with this knowledge, you will be able to seek help for your children in appropriate form and measure—when it is truly needed.

A Homeopathic Scenario

Homeopathic treatment of acute ailments is very swift and decisive. Here is a typical scenario that I see in my professional practice. On Friday, young Tina goes to sleep in a perfectly good mood, looking forward to the weekend because the family is planning to visit her grandparents. Trips like that are always so much fun! Unfortunately, she wakes up the next morning sick. Her parents phone me early in the morning and report that Tina has diarrhea and vomiting, accompanied by severe weakness, a high fever, and cold sweats.

I know Tina pretty well. She's a generally healthy child. After listening to the story and asking a few clarifying questions, I suggest the following plan: her parents will give Tina one pill of the homeopathic remedy *Veratrum album* in a concentration of 200C and then wait for fifteen to twenty minutes. If her condition doesn't improve, they'll immediately take their daughter to the nearest emergency room.

Tina's mother calls me fifteen minutes later to report that Tina felt much better after taking the remedy and has gone to sleep. Among other things, her fever seems to have come down a bit. I suggest letting her sleep and closely monitoring her temperature. I receive another call in about three more hours. Tina feels much better. She has no fever, no nausea, and no diarrhea. She wants to go on the family trip. Although the trip does not ultimately happen, Tina remains fine and is able to attend school on Monday.

Similar scenarios happen in the lives of thousands of families all around the world every day. Some of these children get homeopathy; others are treated with conventional medications. Homeopathic remedies resolve acute problems quickly, often in a matter of minutes or hours. Conventional medications may seem equally impressive at first glance—for instance, if they bring a fever down quickly. But the results are actually very different. Medications suppress a child's symptoms without addressing the root issues that caused them. The conventional approach masks the underlying cause of an illness, frequently leading to more complicated problems for the child in the future.

Restoring Harmony in Your Child's Body

In 1960, author Harry Harrison published *Deathworld*. In this science fiction novel, a gambler named Jason dinAlt is hired to win money for the planet Pyrrus so that its colonists can purchase state-of-the-art weaponry. They need the arms because they are faced with an incredibly hostile ecosystem. Plants and animals on their world constantly develop new ways of killing people. Deadly mutations happen so quickly that anyone who leaves the planet, even for a short vacation, has to undergo extensive weapons training. On return, dinAlt learns that the flora and fauna are so hostile that even Pyrran children must be trained to defend themselves. Inhabitants are so involved in this constant war that they fail to recognize that they are losing it. The population is steadily declining.

There is a great twist at the end. When dinAlt dedicates himself to stopping the carnage, he discovers that the environment has simply been responding to the aggression of the planet's inhabitants. The moment the colonists lay down their weapons, the planet ceases attacking them, and peace and harmony are restored.

Many years ago, I read this book and was impressed by how closely the story line resembles the medical situation in the Western world over the last eighty or ninety years. Since the advent of modern suppressive medications, our population has had to deal with the need to create more drugs due to the emergence of new chronic illnesses that are more difficult to treat, such as allergies, ADHD, autism, obesity, and depression. But drugs—and the way they're dispensed—are partly to blame for their own obsolescence.

Russians have a proverb: teach a fool to bow and he'll break his forehead. One of the most glaring examples of creating a health problem by abusing a potential solution is the uncontrolled use of antibiotics. Without any doubt, the discovery of antibiotics has saved millions of lives. But due to mindless, unnecessary applications of these powerful weapons to relatively benign diseases, a good thing has been turned into a big problem. Microbes "attack." Doctors dispense antibiotics in order to kill the bacteria, not to support the body's natural defenses. Soon the microbes mutate and become drug resistant. Then we feel we must introduce more powerful antibiotics to "counterattack"—and the process goes on and on! Does it remind you of the situation on planet Pyrrus?

Conventional medicine has embraced the belief that the body cannot overcome the adversities of daily life. Doctors prescribe drugs to suppress symptoms. But in the process of suppressing an aggressor, such as a microbe, the body also gets suppressed. After all, the body is made from cells similar to bacteria. Even if the problem is resolved, damage may be done to the body's defense systems. Patients are made weaker, rather than strengthened.

Children with ear infections or sinus infections, for example, generally are given antibiotics every time they get sick. They never develop immunity to infections, so they begin to get sick repeatedly, and then more frequently. Sometimes they become allergic to antibiotics, which can lead to worse systemic reactions, such as asthma.

Wait a minute! Do we really need to use antibiotics as our first recourse, or so often? It is clear that modern science recognizes that the human body can defend itself against microbial attacks—if its defense mechanisms are stimulated using signals the body understands. Consider the smallpox vaccine. Frequently, even strong antibiotics cannot kill the microbe that causes smallpox. But vaccination, a process where you give a dead or weakened form of a microbe to a healthy person, triggers an immune response that protects someone for years from dangerous illnesses like smallpox, rabies, and polio.

Homeopathic remedies stimulate an innate healing response. They can be taken after, and sometimes even before, coming down with an illness. The goal of homeopathic treatment is not to suppress symptoms; rather it's to restore the body's natural defense mechanisms so we can fight against infectious agents on our own—

now and in the future—and win. Because it is extremely effective, homeopathy makes children resilient and less susceptible to disease.

About the American Institute of Homeopathy

Established in 1844, in response to the national need for medical standards, the American Institute of Homeopathy (AIH) was the first professional medical organization in the United States. Our membership comprises medical doctors, osteopathic physicians, dentists, nurse practitioners, and physician assistants. AIH's primary purpose is the improvement and dissemination of knowledge pertaining to homeopathic medicine. The institute has survived the vicissitudes of fortune attendant upon homeopathy and, indeed, upon the whole field of complementary and alternative medicine in the United States, to find itself still extant in a time when the cultural milieu is more welcoming to our practices.

During the second half of the nineteenth century and the first two decades of the twentieth century, homeopathy dominated the medical scene in the United States. Its subsequent decline was dramatic and seemingly sudden. Many opponents of homeopathy claim that its near demise was due to the fact that it is a bogus form of medicine and "simply does not work." But its successes speak for themselves.

That's why homeopathy remained popular in the rest of the world and reemerged with vigor in the United States in the 1970s. Why then did it almost disappear for fifty years? And why are many conventional physicians reluctant to accept it? To answer these questions, we have to look carefully at the history of homeopathy in America.

A Brief History of Homeopathy in America

Since its inception, homeopathy has been firmly grounded in science. When prominent German physician, chemist, and pharmacologist Samuel C. Hahnemann discovered the principles of homeopathy at the end of the eighteenth century, after more than six years of thorough experimental work, his research created a foundation for contemporary biomedicine. During an era of blood-letting, blistering, and purging, he developed a scientifically based and holistic approach to the patient. Despite vehement opposition by the medical establishment, patients appreciated its efficacy immediately.

After enormous success in treating people with scarlet fever and cholera, the practice of homeopathy quickly spread across Europe and to the United States. Unlike *allopathic* (meaning traditional Western) medicine of the period, homeopathy was based in reliable research data and yielded significantly better results. The highway of homeopathy's success has been paved with the gemstones of great discoveries and illuminated by the bright minds of exceptional individuals.

Hans Burch Gram, M.D., brought homeopathy to America in 1825. Born into a family of Danish immigrants in Boston, Gram traveled at the age of eighteen to Copenhagen to attend the Royal Medical and Surgical Institute. After serving as a military surgeon, Gram settled into a general practice and studied homeopathy with one of Hahnemann's students. The second homeopathic doctor in the United States was John Gray, M.D., who was the physician of a prominent businessman whose long-standing digestive problems he could not resolve. When he learned that Gram had cured this patient with homeopathy, Gray met with him to discuss three other difficult cases. These patients were cured too. After that, Gray became a devoted student of homeopathy and later a practitioner. He was an editor of the *American Journal of Homeopathy* and in due course would play an instrumental role in setting up the AIH.

By the early 1830s, the number of American homeopaths had rapidly grown. As with Gray, the field was attractive to many medical doctors. Homeopathy was efficacious and was also underscored by a coherent, meaningful theory based on the experimental data. Some homeopaths were European immigrants. One of these was Constantine Hering, M.D. With his arrival, homeopathy in America received its leader.

Hering was born in Germany on January 1, 1800. He studied medicine at the University of Leipzig under the tutelage of a famous surgeon, Henrich Robbi, M.D., in a period when severe opposition to homeopathy was growing in Europe. Robbi was asked to write a book taking a stand against homeopathy, but he was too busy and so passed the offer on to his beloved student, Hering. In the process, he triggered Hering's enthusiasm.

For the purpose of writing the book, Hering decided to follow a challenge that Hahnemann had included in the Preface of his book *Materia Medica Pura:* "The doctrine [of similars] appeals not only chiefly, but solely to the verdict of experience. . . . Repeat the experiments. Repeat them carefully and accurately, and you will find the doctrine confirmed at every step."[1] *Materia Medica* is an old name for a textbook on pharmacology. He decided to repeat the original experiment with a remedy known as Peruvian bark, which had led Hahnemann to the discovery of homeopathy. Hering was impressed. The results completely proved the principles he'd been invited to condemn. Perhaps needless to say, he never wrote a book ridiculing homeopathy.

In 1821, shortly after this incident, Hering was cured with a "ridiculously minute dose" of homeopathy from a gangrene of the right index finger that he had received during the dissection of a cadaver. The only alternative that had been offered by his conventional physicians was an amputation. In a state of gratitude, Hering wrote, "When the various symptoms of recovery from this terrible affliction began to pervade me, there vanished the last obstacle interposed between my eyes and the rising sun of new healers. The finger is still my own. . . . To Hahnemann who restored . . . the hand, even more the man, body and soul."[2]

Hering also wrote about the excitement he felt after discovering homeopathy: "My enthusiasm grew. I became a fanatic. I went about the country, visited inns, where I got up on tables . . . [to give speeches] about homeopathy. I told people that they were in the hands of cutthroats and murderers. Success came everywhere. I almost thought I could raise the dead."[3]

Impressed with homeopathy, Hering sent his first letter to Hahnemann in 1824. Hahnemann responded with great interest. This started a lifetime exchange of correspondence between these two great men.

Hering graduated medical school in 1826. He then received a commission from the king of Saxony to participate in a botanical and zoological expedition to Surinam, in South America. In Surinam, he became interested in the possible use of deadly snake poisons as remedies. The original experiment—in homeopathy called a *proving*—of the first such snake remedy, *Lachesis muta* (bushmaster snake venom), is surrounded by legend. In 1991, the homeopathic journal *Simillimum* published a translation of Hering's notes. It seems that during the initial stage of dilution of the venom, Hering accidentally ingested a fairly high concentration of it. But like the dedicated researcher he was, while recovering he kept a detailed diary of all the symptoms that resulted from his error. *Lachesis* has subsequently become one of the major homeopathic remedies.

Hering arrived in America by boat, landing on Martha's Vineyard, an island in Massachusetts, in January 1833. With him, he brought a large biological and botanical collection that he later donated to the Academy of Natural Sciences in Philadelphia. It included two large bushmaster snakes, one male (used for the original *Lachesis muta* experiments) and one female. Today, every time a group of homeopaths goes to the Museum of Natural History in Philadelphia, the snakes are proudly displayed.

Hering's colossal contributions to the field of homeopathy include writing the seminal ten-volume work *The Guiding Symptoms of Our Materia Medica* and conducting 104 provings (which are a method for discovering the medicinal qualities of homeopathic drugs). One of these drugs is *Glonoine*, or nitroglycerin, a medication still used to relieve acute cardiac pain.

On April 10, 1835, less than two years after his arrival in the United States, Hering opened the world's first homeopathic school, the North American Academy of the Homeopathic Healing Art, in Allentown, Pennsylvania. All the courses were provided in German. Sadly, the school had to close its doors a mere six years later, because the banker who was handling its endowment made an egregious financial mistake. By that time, however, the academy had trained a core group of homeopathic physicians and educators, who became instrumental in promoting homeopathy throughout the United States.

The founding of the AIH in 1844 was propitious. Three years later, in 1847, partially in response to the incredibly fast development of homeopathy, conventional physicians formed the American Medical Association (AMA). The AMA charter contained a clause that prohibited its members from consulting with homeopaths at the risk of expulsion. The war between homeopathy (the "new school") and allopathic medicine (the "old school") shifted into high gear.

By the mid-1850s, the overwhelming majority of state medical societies (with the exception of the Massachusetts Medical Society) expelled their homeopathic members. In 1856, the AMA banned homeopathic papers from being printed in medical publications. Communication between the two schools of thought ceased. Some situations like this would be considered ridiculous, if they were not so scary. For example, in 1878 a physician was expelled from a local medical society in Connecticut for consulting with a homeopath—his wife!

Nevertheless, despite this opposition from conventional allopathic medicine, homeopathy became extremely popular during the 1850s. About two dozen homeopathic educational institutions were founded in and around that decade. In 1848, a homeopathic medical college was established in Philadelphia. Many of its founders were also founding members of the AIH. In 1869, this college combined with another similar institution to form Hahnemann Medical College.

At the turn of the twentieth century, fifteen thousand physicians described themselves as homeopaths. In June 1900, the AIH celebrated the success of American homeopathy with the public dedication of the Hahnemann Monument in Washington, D.C., a ceremony graced by the presence of President William McKinley and various other dignitaries. This was homeopathy's pinnacle.

However, organized homeopathy was not equipped to deal appropriately with the dramatic changes in society that would soon follow.

One of the major factors leading to a decline of interest in homeopathy in the early twentieth century was the development of the industrialized world. Enormous progress in physics and engineering had resulted in the invention of electric lights, telephones, and automobiles. Physiologist Claude Bernard had described the body as a machine. Society expected medicine to provide simple, mechanical solutions. In addition, due to mass production, the working class grew exponentially. People had to be able to get a quick fix from the doctor and go back to work. Louis Pasteur's germ theory was already well-known. Patented medications came on the market to wipe out germs. Hours for interviews with homeopaths and ample time for recovery became a luxury.

Large pharmaceutical companies were on the rise as a result of the huge profits they made during the Civil War. Yes, homeopathic remedies were more efficacious than patented medicines, and homeopaths were getting better results than medical doctors, but the substantial numbers of "OK" results were convincing enough to draw support from the medical establishment. Society wanted medicine to be simplified, and the drug industry offered the solution in the form of proprietary medications. Single homeopathic medications, by contrast, and with rare exceptions, were nonproprietary as they'd already existed for decades and had become a part of the public domain.

Pharmaceutical companies needed more allopathic physicians to promote their products. Physicians did not need to place an intellectual effort into designing individualized prescriptions. Now all they had to do was to memorize the names of the latest drugs. When the AMA allowed advertisements of proprietary drugs in medical journals, the juggernaut picked up speed.

Another blow to homeopathy came *after* the AMA opened its membership ranks to homeopaths. Interestingly, Dr. McCormack, the man behind this promotion in 1911, stated, "We must admit that we have never fought the homeopath on matters of principle; we fought him because he came into our community and got the business."[4] Younger, less experienced homeopaths got caught up in the wave to prescribe proprietary medications. Combined with the poor quality of homeopathic instruction in schools of the era, this trend was detrimental.

Unfortunately, by the beginning of the twentieth century, a large number of physicians who called themselves homeopaths, including the leaders of the AIH during that period, were no longer adhering to basic principles of homeopathic practice. In 1909, the Carnegie Foundation commissioned a survey on the quality of U.S. medical schools. The Flexner report, as it was known, resulted in closures of a significant number of medical schools, including most homeopathic schools.

Despite everything, homeopathy continued to demonstrate impressive results when it was used appropriately. During the flu epidemic of 1918, the mortality rate among patients treated with homeopathic remedies was less than 1 percent. The mortality rate for patients treated with allopathic medicine was somewhere between 10 percent and 30 percent. A few dedicated individuals realized that homeopathy had to be preserved!

In 1924, Dr. Julia M. Green gathered twelve prominent homeopathic physicians to found a new organization, the American Foundation for Homeopathy (AFH), the main objective of which was to keep homeopathy alive. The AFH created a special bureau to educate laypersons, thereby creating a grassroots preservation movement. Physicians also privately helped keep homeopathy alive as it was being phased out of hospital practice.

During this difficult time period for homeopathy, the AIH continued to function, although the membership ranks were decreasing due to the natural process of elderly homeopaths dying. Very few new members were joining the organization.

World War II gave another significant boost to conventional medications. Doctors who served in the army learned how to use antibiotics, painkillers, and injectables, and they were eager to apply them in their practice. Nonetheless postgraduate homeopathic courses continued. Although it qualified for the status, homeopathy never received recognition as a medical specialization from the AMA.

Yet homeopathy was far from defunct. In January 1960, the AIH established the American Board of Homeotherapeutics to award physicians with the specialty designation Diplomate of Homeotherapeutics (D.Ht.). And some remarkable individuals kept homeopathy alive during the twentieth century. Dr. Marion Belle Rood (1899–1995) of Lapeer, Michigan, is one example. In *The Faces of Homeopathy*, Julian Winston states the following:

> Rood was the only woman in her physics masters program at the University of Michigan in Ann Arbor. She worked on the quantum theory during the 1920s. After two years of teaching mathematics in Tennessee, she attended New York Homeopathic Medical College as the only female student in her class, graduating in 1932.
>
> The stories of Rood are legendary. She lived in a house at the end of the dirt road outside of town. She had neither telephone nor appointments. Her patients would drive up, sit on her porch, and wait. She began at 11 A.M. and would see the patients in the order they had arrived, taking as long as needed for each case. She worked until the last patient was treated, sometimes at 1 A.M. or later. Neighbors often brought snacks for the patients waiting on her porch. . . . Along with Dr. Wyrth Post Baker, she testified before the Senate, to maintain the status of the *Pharmacopoeia* (*Pharmacopoeia* is the book that keeps homeopathic drugs legal in the United States). Rood charged $10 for a visit, raising this to $20, when the *Pharmacopoeia* was again reviewed in the 1980s. She raised and contributed $50,000, which funded the updating of the *US Homoeopathic Pharmacopoeia*.[5]

There were numerous others. However, the format of this handbook does not allow for a detailed description of the many achievements that homeopathic heroes have brought to the altar of homeopathy. The AIH and AFH continued to exist. Postgraduate courses continued to educate physicians about homeopathy. Still the ranks of U.S. homeopaths were depleted until society began changing its attitudes in the 1970s. A new generation of physicians was participating in the search for better answers to promote healing. Many people desired natural alternatives and became more health conscious.

An intriguing benefit of homeopathy's going "underground" in the United States for decades in the twentieth century is that American homeopathy is practiced in a classical style. The few people who did carry it on were true to Hahnemann's original model. They were purists because *classical homeopathy* is the most efficient homeopathy. It works best. So even though the homeopathic schools and hospitals closed, the discipline flourished.

High classical standards of true Hahnemannian homeopathy have been restored by the efforts of many enthusiasts. Classical homeopaths of recent years have been able to demonstrate good results when treating different acute and chronic conditions that conventional, or allopathic, medicine has been unable to heal, such as autism, post-traumatic stress disorder (PTSD), chronic asthma, chronic sinusitis, and irritable bowel syndrome.

Throughout all these years, the AIH has remained active in promoting high professional and ethical standards of homeopathic practice. Currently, the American professional homeopathic community is strong. Various homeopathic organizations are working together to make homeopathy more accessible. We hope to see full-time homeopathic schools and clinics reemerge in the near future.

A Note to Parents on Working Together

I have been practicing homeopathy for over twenty years, and I have learned an important lesson: different people appreciate different methods of treatment. There are many folks out there who love homeopathy. They simply see how much sense it makes and embrace it. There are other folks who reject homeopathy flat out and won't even consider it.

Here's the rub. Often someone from the first group is coparenting a child with someone from the second group. This situation can create friction. (It's reminiscent of the ridiculous and outmoded professional rivalry between the AMA and the AIH.) Frequently,

I've had to stop consultations and refer my patients to other, more conventional health care providers because one of the parents comes in and says that he or she won't allow "this kind" of treatment. All parents want the best for their children, but sometimes couples see things very differently. For the benefit of their children, they need to learn to work as a team.

Should we expect everyone to be on the same page and choose homeopathy as a first treatment option? My answer is simple: No, we can't! On a superficial level, homeopathy appears to challenge mainstream scientific principles. You may have heard that homeopathic remedies are highly diluted, for instance. How could anything so diluted be useful? There is no trace of a substance in them! Discussions with skeptics usually end at this point. (See Chapter Two for a detailed explanation.) But in fact, such dilution in homeopathic remedies has been proven to be more effective.

Major peer-reviewed medical journals have published articles about the success of homeopathy in double-blind, placebo-controlled clinical research studies. But my faith in homeopathy has also been generated from many direct experiences of watching it work in a wide range of circumstances. A bee stings a child in the neck and it begins to swell. One dose of a homeopathic remedy can resolve this issue on the spot. Small cures such as this are everyday occurrences in my professional practice. In addition, as a devoted father of two daughters, who are now eighteen and twenty, I've faced scary situations when my children suddenly got very sick in the middle of the night. In many, many instances, homeopathy was able to cure their ailments.

As a parent, you know how difficult it is to see your child suffering. What to do?! What to do?! I will never forget what my own wife used to say when this happened for a few years after we had our first child: "We need to call a *real* doctor!" This statement used to drive me crazy. "I *am* a real doctor!" I'd answer. "You know what I mean," she'd go on. "What if our daughter has something serious?"

Although it took me a while to show my wife and the rest of our family how effective homeopathy was, ultimately they were persuaded by direct experiences. At one and a half, our eldest daughter contracted measles, which in Russia, where we were living at the time, was considered a relatively benign condition. As a family physician, I knew the symptoms well—and she had them all. She had a typical rash that was slowly spreading over her body. She also had a high fever, had a dry cough, and was acting tearful and clingy. So I knew exactly what remedy to give her. Measles is a viral illness and antibiotics don't help it much. There really was no choice of how to treat my daughter other than homeopathy.

I shared this information with my wife, who was growing progressively more anxious. The "we need to call a real doctor" comment surfaced very quickly. In reply, I said, "OK. I hear your concern. We'll ask the pediatrician to make a house call. But let's make a deal. If the doctor prescribes antibiotics, you'll give me twelve hours to treat our daughter with homeopathy first, before we use it." My wife agreed.

The pediatrician came at the end of the day. She was a nice, caring, middle-aged woman, who, after examining our daughter, said that there were no signs of significant bronchitis or pneumonia yet, but it would be good to start antibiotics "prophylactically," meaning as a preventive measure. We took the prescription, and after a short argument in which I reminded my wife of everything we had discussed, I was "allowed" to administer a homeopathic remedy. Once I did, my daughter's fever shot up, the rash spread all over her body in the span of just a few hours, and then the fever disappeared. She went to sleep peacefully and woke up the next morning looking like a cute little cheetah cub—covered in tiny red patches characteristic of this illness—but happy, with a good appetite, and without a fever. In a few days, the illness was gone.

To me this example illustrates a few important points:

- Fear frequently drives us to make wrong or hasty decisions.
- We often turn to our arsenal of powerful medications too soon.
- A very prompt curative result is possible after using homeopathy.
- Opposition from a skeptical mate can be overcome.

If your mate does not share your views on homeopathy, please ensure that he or she reads the following message.

In this book, I do *not* advocate abandoning conventional medicine. Millions of people are alive because of the success of allopathic treatments. Every day, scores of people are helped by it. But there are many gray areas where conventional medicine is useless or can only offer treatments that have more risks than benefits.

I *do* suggest that homeopathy can and should be considered a first line of defense in treating childhood diseases. In an emergency, you'll always have the option to give a sick child one dose of a homeopathic remedy on the way to the doctor or to the emergency room.

What I'm asking of you, ladies and gentlemen, is to give homeopathy a chance. Please be reasonable. Speak with each other and do some research. Read the first three chapters of this book, which explain the history of homeopathy and its principles. Consider whether or not this form of medicine makes sense to you. Then arrive at a mutual plan of action, one that is comfortable for both of you, and stick to it.

More than anything, your children need you, their parents, to function as a team. If, after studying the subject, you don't feel that homeopathy makes sense, that's fine. At least you gave it your best consideration and made a decision *together*.

How to Use This Book

Written under the auspices of the AIH, this handbook will provide you with a proven method to treat many acute and chronic conditions. Homeopathy is a safe, effective way to stimulate the body's innate healing response and restore your child's natural health.

Part One, "An Introduction to Homeopathic Treatment for Children," offers a foundation of knowledge about homeopathy. Here you can find valuable information about its main principles, its benefits and risks, how homeopathic remedies are prepared, and how to work with a practitioner. We'll look into a few myths and controversies, too.

Most children are healthy. In general, all they need in order to heal is the kind of gentle guidance that's provided by homeopathy. This approach allows our children to draw upon their own powerful defenses, and as a result it makes their immune systems more resilient. Best of all, with homeopathy, your children will have no more side effects and no more allergic reactions from medicine.

In Part Two, "Treating Acute Health Problems," we are going to show you ways to make your children strong and healthy by using homeopathy successfully to treat their everyday ailments—those that don't require heroic measures—as well as their acute ailments, those that can be permanently cured. To find the right remedy, you need to know what changes—characteristic to your child—have been caused by the illness. In acute conditions, changes are obvious because they are new and strong. A relatively limited number of remedies are useful, and some are specific to a particular situation. For example, *Cocculus* and *Tabacum* are most frequently indicated for car sickness. Here you'll learn about sixty-three remedies that all parents should have in their medicine chests. Then we'll list common conditions and the remedies that most often cure them.

In Part Three, "Treating Chronic Mental Health and Physical Problems," we'll evaluate homeopathic options for the successful treatment of four chronic mental health problems that have been plaguing the children in our society in recent decades: ADHD, anxiety, autism, and depression. Homeopathy produces excellent results for these and other chronic issues. Then we'll explore the process of effective treatment for five chronic physical ailments: allergies, asthma, eczema, sinusitis, and obesity. Identifying the correct remedy for a chronic condition is a different and more complicated process then finding a remedy for an acute ailment. You'll require the assistance of a homeopath to achieve the necessary precision.

In chronic illnesses, the whole child, with all of his or her individual characteristics, must be thoroughly evaluated. Changes can be very subtle and the choice of remedy becomes laborious. This type of prescribing is known as *constitutional treatment*, because the homeopath attempts to find the remedy that will initiate a healing process of the entire child.

After reading the first three explanatory chapters, you'll be ready to begin using homeopathy on a daily basis to improve the health of your children. It's also a good idea to read through the book from beginning to end at least once, just to get an overview of the essential guidelines of homeopathic prescribing. Then keep the book on a shelf in your kitchen or bedroom, and refer to different sections as needed. In these pages, you can quickly find the answers to almost all of the health problems your children might have. It is designed to be the main tool in helping your children achieve optimum wellness. We hope it provides you and your family with a sense of security and comfort for many years to come.

Part One

An Introduction to Homeopathic Treatment for Children

Chapter One

The Basic Principles of Homeopathy

Without a doubt, this is the most important chapter in this book. In it, you'll learn what homeopathy is and how it differs from conventional Western, or *allopathic*, medicine. I'd wager you're probably just looking to learn about a few homeopathic remedies so you can help your children, and I promise that you'll find such information in these pages. Yet homeopathy differs enormously from conventional medicine. So before you can set out on a course of homeopathic healing, you need to understand a few significant details. Otherwise you may be as astonished and disbelieving as Tim's parents were.

As happens frequently in my homeopathic practice, I saw Tim after his parents had already tried every single conventional approach offered to them by dermatologists. Tim was thirteen and he had an awful case of eczema. Lesions had spread all over his body, most looking like various stages of poison ivy, and they were, as Tim put it, "very ugly." The itching was enormous. Luckily, he only had a few marks on his face.

Tim and his parents felt devastated. This good-looking, intelligent boy couldn't socialize, as he was afraid that other kids would make fun of him. He avoided going to the beach, swimming in the pool, or playing sports. After all, what if another student saw his embarrassing lesions while he was changing in the locker room? His parents were also concerned that the eczema wouldn't get better no matter what they did. They'd heard from dermatologists that kids usually "outgrow" eczema. But it hadn't happened so far.

As far as homeopathy is concerned, the severity of skin lesions doesn't matter as long as the patient is otherwise healthy. In our initial consultation, I determined that Tim was. I therefore knew I simply had to find the correct remedy. One dose of that exact remedy would probably take care of everything. Of course, this was easy for me to say. The parents told me honestly that if not for the utter failure of conventional treatments, including steroids, they would never have considered bringing their son to a homeopath. In the end, they only came because a mutual friend recommended me as trustworthy.

After taking a look at Tim's lesions, I conducted a full homeopathic interview. The questions I asked were seemingly strange. I was mostly interested in what made his rash feel better or worse, and in what made Tim different from other people. I wanted to know his eating and sleeping habits and about his relationship with the weather, animals, and people. I needed to understand what made this particular child with eczema different from everyone else with the same diagnosis. In addition, I needed to match the set of symptoms that Tim was then exhibiting with the set of symptoms that had been triggered in healthy volunteers by a homeopathic substance during initial research that was conducted to understand its curative properties. That's how a homeopath carefully picks a remedy.

After about an hour and a half, I made a decision. I gave Tim a 200C dose of a homeopathic remedy called *Rhus toxicodendron*. He dissolved the sugary pellet under his tongue and told me he liked its sweetness. I explained to his parents that I'd given him a preparation of poison ivy that had been diluted 10^{400} (that is, 10 to the four hundredth power) times. Tim's father was a chemist. He said, "That's crazy. Nothing diluted this much can work." He was also surprised that I wanted Tim to take a pill only once. Both parents seemed disappointed that there was nothing else I was willing to offer. Nevertheless they didn't have a choice.

I asked Tim's parents to wait six to eight weeks and then come in for a follow-up appointment. Two months later, they brought Tim back. The rash was gone! Tim was so happy that he decided to become a homeopath when he grew up. They reported that about five days after taking the *Rhus*, Tim complained of an increased rash and itching. But a few days later, the itching subsided and the lesions started to disappear. The skin on the upper parts of his body healed first, and then the rash completely went away.

Interestingly, not all cases of eczema would have responded to *Rhus*. To the contrary, I've successfully prescribed many other remedies for the same skin condition. In homeopathy, we treat the individual patient rather than suppress the symptoms of a disease. Like Tim, his parents were thrilled with the results of homeopathy. But they still wondered if we should give Tim more of the remedy, just to make sure he would be fine in the future. I explained to them that it wasn't necessary or even useful. He was cured.

What Is Homeopathy?

Homeopathy is a medical approach that's defined by the principle of *similars*: "like cures like." Its practitioners use small quantities of highly diluted substances that in larger quantities would provoke the same symptoms they intend to cure. In the case of Tim, for instance, we employed heavily diluted poison ivy to heal an itchy skin rash. The idea is to give the body's own healing process a tiny boost. All forms of medicine that don't follow this principle are considered *allopathy*.[1]

In homeopathy, we appreciate symptoms as being the language in which the body speaks to us. They show us that the body is struggling to externalize the potential damage that a deep-seated illness could do at the body's core. If we're seeing various external symptoms, we can be fairly certain that deep damage hasn't been done yet. If these stop, we can assume that either the individual is cured or the illness has reached deeper to the core level.

In allopathy, symptoms are viewed as *being* the illness, rather than as an attempt to heal, which is why conventional doctors believe they must be suppressed. By contrast, homeopathy views the body's expression of symptoms as a healthy mechanism. For this reason, homeopaths treat a patient's set of symptoms with remedies that would cause a similar set of symptoms if taken in sufficient quantity by a healthy person. Like cures like.

The Principle of Similars

Samuel Hahnemann was an extraordinarily intelligent and multi-talented man. Born April 10, 1755, into the family of a poor German porcelain painter, he had to work from a young age. At twelve, he was already tutoring Greek. Later on, he became a prolific writer, translator, doctor, chemist, and pharmacologist. Once he presented a thesis in Latin at the University of Leipzig. During this presentation, Hahnemann apparently quoted sources in eight original languages, including Hebrew and Arabic.

A tragic misconception about homeopathy is that it has no scientific basis. This statement couldn't be further from the truth. As you read on, I'm sure you'll appreciate how much Hahnemann has done for modern biomedical science. He introduced many ground-breaking ideas into medical practice. Hahnemann discovered homeopathy at age thirty-five by conducting a series of experiments on himself. In the process, he invented reliable research methods. Prior to that, he was already deeply involved with nutrition and noninvasive healing. We're talking about the 1700s here! Clearly a man way ahead of his time, without any doubt, Hahnemann deserves recognition as being the father of modern scientifically based medicine, both homeopathic and conventional.

Hahnemann's discovery of homeopathy began when he was translating a book on pharmacology that described Peruvian bark, a preparation made from a tree that was highly effective in treating malaria. As medicine in his era had no scientific basis, the only explanation offered by the textbook for Peruvian bark's curative effect was that it had the capacity to upset the stomach. It was a cockamamie time for medicine. The most respected theory of the era was the *doctrine of signatures*, which a German mystic named Jacob Boehme had popularized in two books, *Aurora* and *The Signature of All Things*, more than a century earlier.

The doctrine of signatures was a purely philosophical notion until Boehme's predecessor, the alchemist Paracelsus, had applied it to medicine. It postulated that certain features of a plant carry indications of its medicinal use. For example, plants with yellow roots or flowers (yellow signature) were supposed to cure jaundice. Plants impregnated with the color red (red signature) were considered to be beneficial for blood disorders. The hue of iris resembled bruises, so that's what the plant was used to treat. Also the shape of plants played an important role in determining their uses.

Hahnemann couldn't accept the textbook's silly explanation for why Peruvian bark worked so well. He decided to take the preparation himself and find out what would happen. After a few repeated doses of Peruvian bark, he developed symptoms that closely resembled the symptoms of malaria. These subsided shortly after discontinuation of the medication. Hahnemann described this experiment in a footnote to the translation, which was published in 1790. Six years later, after a continual literature search and further experimentation, Hahnemann published a landmark article, "Essay on a New Principle for Ascertaining the Curative Powers of Drugs." In this piece, he proclaimed the discovery of a curative law of nature: *Similia similibus curentur* (like cures like).

You were introduced to the principle of similars in the story about Tim's eczema. Let's look at another real present-day example to see how it operates. Yellow-jasmine poisoning causes severe weakness with significant heaviness in the back of the head, heavy eyelids, and chills running up and down the back.[2] The homeopathic preparation of this flower, a remedy called *Gelsemium*, has shown to be very helpful for treating the flu in people who develop the same set of symptoms.

Superficially, it might seem as though the use of the conventional drug Ritalin for the treatment of attention deficit–hyperactivity disorder (ADHD) follows the principle of similars. Ritalin is a stimulant given to children who are restless to calm them. But the way the medication is typically used actually doesn't correlate with our natural law.

For a medication to be suitable for a specific patient, other individual characteristics must be present, besides the ones that everyone exhibits. In the case of ADHD, as a common symptom is restlessness, we would look elsewhere. The same remedy won't work for everyone. Furthermore, remedies need to be homeopathically prepared—diluted and activated. This process is described in detail in Chapter Two.

Another interesting modern example demonstrating the principle of similars is the conventional allergy elimination technique. First, an allergist conducts a series of tests to find the allergen that's affecting someone. Then this same allergen is given to that individual in significantly smaller and smaller concentrations until the allergy goes away. Many children and adults have benefited from the application of this technique.

Interestingly, in the same year that Hahnemann published his seminal paper on homeopathy, British physician Edward Jenner published a paper on vaccination. He noticed that milkmaids never got sick with smallpox, a terrible, deadly infectious disease. But most of them had experienced cowpox, an illness benign to humans. Jenner cleverly suspected that milkmaids were protected from smallpox by the similar illness. He therefore decided to inoculate people with cowpox to protect them from smallpox. In Latin, *vacca* means "cow." His idea worked perfectly. As a result, 1796 gave birth to two great medical discoveries, both of which incorporated the principle of similars.

Testing New Remedies

During his research on Peruvian bark, Hahnemann invented an experimental method for finding new remedies and investigating their qualities. He called this process a *prüfung*, meaning a "test." In English, it's known as a *proving*. Original provings were conducted using alcohol-based tinctures of various substances. Essentially, he took the substance and then experienced a set of symptoms, which he recorded in great detail. Healthy volunteers, or *provers*, also received repeated doses of the substance in question and then would describe all the symptoms they experienced.

Obviously, people have varying levels of sensitivity to particular substances and therefore develop different sets of symptoms, depending on their individual dispositions. A few of the provers were highly sensitive to a particular substance and would develop hundreds, often thousands, of symptoms. Other provers weren't sensitive to it at all.

As mentioned in the Introduction, the systematic summary of everyone's combined symptoms is called *Materia Medica,* an old name for a textbook on pharmacology. It's a collection of symptoms experienced by a pool of provers and also symptoms that arose during cases of accidental poisoning. At a later point, symptoms cured by the remedy that weren't in the original provings were also included in *Materia Medica.*

Provings were a prototype for the first phase in contemporary pharmacological studies of conventional drugs. There's a major difference between a proving and a *phase I study,* however. Phase I studies are designed to establish side effects. Homeopathic remedies don't have any "side" effects. All effects discovered in a proving are used to match a particular substance as closely as possible with the symptoms of a particular ill person. When a perfect match—in homeopathic parlance, the *simillimum* (meaning "similar" in Latin)—is found, a remedy is administered to that sick person in order to stimulate a cure.

Double-blind, placebo-controlled homeopathic provings occurred as early as the first part of the 1800s, whereas the first placebo-controlled study published by conventional medical researchers dates back to a 1948 trial conducted by the Medical Research Council on the use of streptomycin to treat pulmonary tuberculosis. The term *double blind* means that neither the participants nor the researchers in a study know which substance specific participants are receiving. *Placebo-controlled* indicates that an active substance—a medication of any kind—is being compared with a neutral substance, such as a sugar pill. Both requirements ensure that the results of an experiment are nonbiased.

Homeopaths instituted another important research design feature: the *multicenter study*. The importance of multicenter research is that it eliminates the influence of unforeseen variables, such as the character of a regional population and human error. If results are duplicated when conducting the same research in more than one location, that verifies that those results are extremely reliable and accurate. The first multicenter study of a homeopathic remedy (*Belladonna*) was conducted in 1906, whereas the first multicenter study of an allopathic drug was conducted in 1944.

I only present such facts to help you understand how the two hundred–yearlong feud between conventional physicians and homeopaths has translated into ignorance about homeopathy's scientific underpinnings. Unfortunately, our allopathic colleagues don't usually realize how deeply rooted homeopathy is in objective measures. Homeopathic prescribing is based on experimental data received from healthy humans. Its practice is rooted in precise and rational scientific observations.

During Hahnemann's research and professional practice, he continually refined his understanding of homeopathy and his methods. For a long time, Hahnemann used fairly concentrated tinctures of substances. For an unknown reason, he started to dilute remedies in proportions of 1:10 (called *decimal*, from the Latin word for ten, and marked with the letter X) or 1:100 (called *centesimal*, from the Latin word for one hundred, and marked with the letter C). Between each of a series of *dilutions*, he hit the tube against a thick book ten to twenty times. He called this process *potentization*.

Hahnemann believed that vigorous shaking helped to extract healing energy from the active substance in the remedy: a vital force that could produce a response in a patient's vital force. Frankly, we don't yet have a better explanation. But we do know that he discovered that higher serial dilutions provide deeper and longer-lasting results than lower serial dilutions. He didn't "dream up" or theorize these results. He just followed the data he was objectively collecting from the numerous patients he treated. It wasn't unusual for him to administer remedies diluted 10^{400} times (200C) or more.

Today the majority of contemporary homeopaths from North America, Great Britain, and India use *ultramolecular dilutions*, as Hahnemann did. But, interestingly, a large group of homeopaths from other countries successfully employ remedies that contain discernible concentrations of original source materials. These remedies are still prepared by dilution with potentization, but they are much less diluted. Consequently, when they're taken, they require significantly more frequent repetition than higher dilutions—for instance, taking two to three doses a day for a duration of a month or more, as opposed to taking one dose every few months, or even years, for ultramolecular dilutions.

The concept of ultramolecular dilutions, although significant, is not central to homeopathy. It's more important to remember that during the process of serial dilution, the tube is vigorously shaken, or *succussed*, between each step. How remedies are manufactured will be explained in detail in Chapter Two.

Extremely Safe and Gentle

Physicians are taught in medical school that it's better to do nothing than to take an action that might harm a patient. This is the guiding principle of medicine and has been for twenty-five hundred years. According to legend, Hippocrates, the renowned Ancient Greek physician known as the *father of medicine*, was already telling his students, "First do no harm." Unfortunately, we know too well from past experience that conventional medications almost always produce side effects—some mild and some severe. A cold remedy can make you drowsy. An antibiotic can upset your stomach, cause severe allergies, or destroy important friendly bacteria in your gut. We often accept minor side effects as the "price we must pay."

Homeopathic remedies are nontoxic because they are highly diluted substances. In addition, they have no side effects, although in some sensitive children certain symptoms may appear. Occasionally, I'll receive a call from a frantic mother whose child has just ingested half a container of a 30C potency remedy. Each container holds about seventy pellets. Anyone familiar with basic math can understand that even if taken at once, the entire contents couldn't possibly cause any complications. The active ingredient in a 30C remedy has been diluted 10^{60}. That's a ten with sixty zeros following it ($10 \times 10 \times 10 \ldots$ sixty times over).

Homeopathy is safer than conventional medicine. Look, you receive instructions on correct usage when either an allopathic doctor or a homeopath prescribes medication to you. The crucial difference is that if you correctly follow the instructions when you take a homeopathic remedy, nothing bad is going to happen. But even if you correctly follow a doctor's instructions when taking a conventional drug, it could have side effects.

The principle of safety has played a defining role in my own life. It was a cold Russian winter in 1984, and I was working as a family physician in Moscow. A doctor in our clinic called in sick, so I agreed to cover her home visits. It was a busy day for me, full of cases of common colds and bronchitis. As one of the addresses belonged to a close friend of mine, I left this visit for the end of my tour. It would be so nice to meet him and talk about the American science fiction and jazz music we both liked! Finally, I was at his home. I rang the bell. A beautiful young lady opened the door, the patient. She turned out to be my friend's sister, Natasha. I never knew he had such a beautiful sister!

After examining Natasha, I diagnosed her with a mild case of bronchitis and offered her a few choices. She could take herbal expectorants, conventional medication, or homeopathy. She'd heard homeopathy was very good and was surprised that a local family physician knew about it. In Russia, homeopaths are highly respected and usually expensive. She was eager to try it. Because I liked her and she was my friend's sister, I volunteered to go and fetch the remedy for her. She was instructed to take one pellet three times a day. During our follow-up appointment, Natasha admitted that the pellets were so little and tasted so delicious that eventually she took all those remaining at once.

The results were amazing. Whatever I gave her worked well. She was cured. We got married a few months later and we're still together. Did Natasha's treatment have any side effects? Actually, it did. We now have two beautiful daughters.

Hahnemann was firm on the principle of giving a single remedy to a patient at one time. Throughout his life, he fought against the practice of polypharmacy, or prescribing numerous medications to the same patient, a problem that persists in allopathic medicine. Adverse reactions to medications must often be attributed to drug interactions. Two hundred years of experience have shown that homeopathic clinicians who follow the principle of using a single remedy receive much better and longer-lasting results.

Of course, finding the special remedy for a special person can sometimes be difficult. But the results are spectacular. Soon you'll see for yourself.

Consistently Proven Effective

The foremost benefit of homeopathy is its efficacy. In fact, the primary reason homeopaths are enthusiastic about what we do is that we are privileged to witness the miracle of a complete cure every day. Frankly, we never get used to it. Even after practicing homeopathy for more than twenty years, I'm still amazed at how quickly the human body can recover from a seemingly dangerous condition after the administration of a lone tiny pellet. At conferences and social gatherings, whenever several homeopaths are in the room, there's an endless exchange of stories about the numerous "little" cures they've seen for acute conditions, such as hives, colic, and poison ivy, and the "big," amazing cures they've seen for severe chronic illnesses, such as asthma and ADHD.

Its consistent success rate was the most important factor in making homeopathy popular in the early 1800s, and it has kept the practice of homeopathy alive in the United States since then, despite conventional medicine's opposition to its principles and methods. Of course, every homeopathic practitioner has experienced failures, yet our outstanding success in curing both children and adults motivates us to continue our efforts to find the perfect remedy for those patients we couldn't help right away.

Samuel Hahnemann became a medical celebrity in 1799 due to an early success. Only three years after homeopathy's official discovery, an epidemic of scarlet fever swept Germany. Children were the main victims of the illness, which is a severe form of strep throat. Hahnemann achieved such impressive results in the treatment and prevention of this deadly illness that soon many allopathic physicians adopted his new approach and began praising homeopathy. The outcome was staggering. Ten physicians gave the homeopathic remedy *Belladonna* to 1,646 children for prophylaxis, or preventive treatment, and they reported that only 123 developed the illness, whereas the morbidity rate in the untreated population surged as high as 90 percent! Subsequently, the protomedicus of Prussia, a public health official comparable to our surgeon general, declared the remedy effective, and the government made the use of *Belladonna* for the prevention of scarlet fever mandatory. Today the scope of this decision would be similar to having the U.S. government recommend homeopathy for the treatment of cancer or AIDS.

From its inception, homeopathy has been able to treat epidemics with impressive results, making the approach popular worldwide. In *The Logic of Figures,* first published in 1900, Thomas Bradford, M.D., a homeopath and historian, compared success rates from allopathic therapeutics with those from homeopathy. Here are some interesting statistics that he put together:

- In 1813, following the defeat of Napoleon's army by the Russians, retreating French troops carried an epidemic of typhoid fever through Europe. When the epidemic hit Leipzig, Hahnemann saw 180 cases of typhus. He cured all but two, representing a 1 percent mortality rate. Conventional physicians reported a 30 percent mortality rate.

- In the European cholera epidemic of 1831–1832, homeopathic hospitals had 7 to 10 percent mortality rates, whereas conventional physicians saw rates of 40 to 80 percent. As a result, a law forbidding the practice of homeopathy in Austria was dropped.
- In 1854, cholera broke out in London. The House of Commons asked for a report comparing various methods of treatment. Initially, homeopathic figures weren't included. According to the report, the mortality rate for patients under allopathic care was 59 percent. In response to an inquiry by the House of Lords, statistics for patients under homeopathic care were then provided. The mortality rate was only 9 percent.
- During the 1850s, several epidemics of yellow fever hit the southern United States. Today we know that mosquitoes transmit this disease. William Osler, a prominent physician of that era and author of the famous book *Systems of Medicine*, reported that the allopathic mortality rate from yellow fever was 15 to 85 percent. Homeopaths reported a mortality rate between 6 and 7 percent. In a similar epidemic in 1878, the mortality in New Orleans as reported by allopathic physicians was 50 percent. Homeopaths reported mortality of 6 percent for 1,945 cases.
- Children have always been easy targets for severe infectious diseases, and one of the most deadly of these was diphtheria. Although diphtheria was eventually eliminated by the advent of widespread vaccination, before then it was difficult to treat, as it rarely had the same presentation. Almost every case was a life-or-death proposition. Records from 1862 to 1864 in Broome County, New York, indicate an 84 percent mortality rate for patients given conventional medicine and only a 16 percent mortality rate for patients given homeopathy. Individualization of the homeopathic treatment was the most crucial factor in its success.
- Another devastating childhood disease is polio. Before the polio vaccine, this illness used to spread in epidemics, paralyzing and killing huge numbers of children. The most memorable outbreak was the infamous polio epidemic of the 1950s. An American homeopath, Arthur Grimmer, M.D., and an Argentinean homeopath, Francisco Eizayaga, M.D., both reported excellent results

from using homeopathy to prevent and treat polio prior to the introduction of the vaccine.

• In 1996, the Homeopathic Medicine Research Group, which was formed by the European Union to determine the effectiveness of homeopathy, conducted a large study. It's important to know that scientists skeptical of homeopathy were involved in the design of the study. The study analyzed outcomes from seventeen clinical trials on a total of 2,001 subjects and showed that homeopathy was more effective than a placebo. There was only a slim probability (0.027 percent) that this result was due to chance.

The U.S. Centers for Disease Control and Prevention (CDC) estimate that 10 to 20 percent of Americans come down with the flu annually. Children are two to three times more likely than adults to get sick, and children frequently spread the virus to others. Although most people recover, the CDC estimates that more than 100,000 people in the U.S. are hospitalized, and about 36,000 people die from the flu and its complications every year. Taking statistics into account, homeopathy is a significant untapped resource.

The flu pandemic of 1918–1919 is still remembered for its devastating death toll. Considered the worst epidemic in U.S. history, with 600,000 people dead, it took the lives of 20 to 40 million people worldwide. In 1921, in a long article about the epidemic, the *Journal of the American Institute of Homeopathy* reported that in Dayton, Ohio, the overall mortality rate of flu patients was 28 percent, whereas in 26,000 cases of flu treated homeopathically, patients had a mortality rate of only 1 percent. Hahnemann College in Philadelphia reported a similar figure for their homeopathic treatment of flu in 26,795 cases that year. Similar statistics came from other homeopathic physicians across the country. Flu season typically lasts from November to March. The media-generated panic that surrounds it each year keeps the memories of the earlier disaster alive.

Cases When Homeopathy Won't Work

Homeopathic treatment doesn't work in situations where structural damage has been done to a patient's body, cases such as genetic disorders, birth defects, and other profound physical conditions (for example, side effects from conventional medication or certain types of injuries). In other words, a condition has an *obvious* cause that may or may not be reparable—but if so, only by some means other than homeopathy.

Genetic Disorders and Birth Defects

Homeopathy cannot work if someone has a genetic disorder that's resulted in significant physical or emotional and mental deficiencies. For instance, children with Down's syndrome have multiple health issues. Although many symptoms can be relieved with homeopathy, defects related to intellectual functioning and structural changes of the cartilage cannot be removed. The same is true of other genetic disorders. They are inbuilt.

Pregnant women who consume significant amounts of alcohol or illicit drugs can damage their babies in the womb. These irreversible defects can be quite significant. Interestingly, when attempts are made to treat these children homeopathically, at first there's often a significant improvement in different levels of functioning. But eventually, it trails off. The next prescription usually results in a less-intense and shorter-lived response.

Side Effects of Medication

Frequently, it's impossible to treat the side effects of a conventional drug with homeopathy. But there's a way around the problem.

Imagine that someone comes to the emergency room with a knife sticking out of his thigh and says, "Listen, Doc. You have to help me. But you cannot touch the knife!" Although it would be possible to give the guy painkillers, that type of care would be silly.

To close the case, all you need to do is remove the knife and sew up the wound.

In the instance of treating side effects, my advice is to discuss possibly changing the medication with the doctor who prescribed it.

To be fair, I must admit that some homeopaths claim success in treating side effects of allopathic medications. At least one book has been published on this subject. Still, the proposition doesn't make as much sense as changing medications. Doctors have many drugs of the same type to choose from and can usually adjust their treatments.

Now, of course, an even more reasonable solution is to try to cure an illness with homeopathy rather than conventional means. If you succeed, then your child won't need allopathic medication. But is this true for every illness? What can homeopathy do for terrible chronic diseases, like cancer and AIDS, which don't spare children?

Advances have been made in the homeopathic approach to life-threatening, chronic illnesses. However, conventional physicians have been increasingly successful at saving and prolonging the lives of patients with cancer and AIDS. A significant amount of money has been directed toward the research and development of medications in these areas. Thousands of dedicated physicians and scientists have been working on saving people's lives. We cannot disregard these facts! As a parent, you should always consult with experts in the field before making a critical, life-altering decision.

Reversible Structural Problems

A few years ago, I received a referral patient from a famous homeopath. Noel, a slightly obese woman in her late fifties to early sixties, had been seen by this homeopath three times without success. She complained of excruciating pain in her right shoulder, and her story was quite remarkable. Noel claimed that while she was asleep, her husband, also very large, had rolled over in his sleep, pressed on her chest, and dislocated her right collarbone, thus causing all her subsequent pain.

Every conventional specialist possible saw her. Numerous imaging studies, including an MRI, had been performed. They found nothing. As happens very frequently when doctors don't find answers, Noel was pronounced anxious, depressed, or perhaps psychotic. As a result, she was placed on many painkillers, mood stabilizers, and antidepressants. The list of her medications was long and scary. Certainly, she had many side effects from them, too. Although Noel *knew* that she was right, the doctors' studies just didn't support her claim.

Noel went to an acupuncturist. No results. Finally, she located the famous homeopath. He prescribed a few remedies for her with no effect and also decided that the woman was probably psychotic. That's when I came in handy, for I am a psychiatrist as well as a homeopath. In this case, I made the perfect second opinion.

Noel came to see me along with her husband. The first thing I noticed was that they both were very honest, normal people, and Noel was suffering a lot. After taking a thorough history, I was convinced that there was no evidence of mental illness. I believed Noel's story. I also knew something that the conventional physicians refuse to admit to their patients, which is that there are *osteopathic* physicians. These doctors are specially trained to diagnose and treat structural changes, even if they are very minute.

I sent Noel to an excellent osteopath, who also saw nothing in the tests. But an osteopathic examination showed that her collarbone did move just a tiny bit. In an area so rich with nerve endings, this minute displacement was causing Noel an enormous amount of pain. The osteopath adjusted the problem. Literally, after the very first visit, Noel felt much better. For the first time in many years, her pain was diminishing! In three to four weeks, she was off most of her medication. She was cured!

This case illustrates a few important points. First, it proves— yet again—that our collective knowledge has many limitations, even when we use modern technology. Second, if there is an *apparent* cause of an illness, it has to be removed. Third, do not give up on your convictions about your family's health. If you know why your child is ill, pursue the line of treatment that can remove the cause. Furthermore, medical miracles can happen. I know, for example, that osteopathic physicians adjust severely displaced collarbones in newborns. The results look like a miracle, but they're not. There are many other health care providers, both alternative and conventional, who can treat your child. Of course, I've seen many so-called miracles that happened with homeopathy.

A Holistic Approach

Homeopathy uses a holistic approach. An allopath looks at a patient in segments, as if under a microscope, and frequently forgets about the person as a whole organism. A homeopath looks at a patient through two lenses: a telescopic lens, to see the person's entire health picture, and a microscopic lens, to distinguish what makes this person unique. When we look at people as unified beings with a telescopic perspective, we begin to understand their true level of health. Understanding levels of health is important. We need to know how healthy or sick we are so that we'll know what to expect from our treatment—homeopathic or otherwise—and what various symptoms indicate.

How frequently have you heard about someone with a serious illness who was told by doctors ten years earlier that he had less than a year to live? I'm guessing often. At least, I have. I used to laugh at scenes in movies and books, where a doctor somberly informs a patient, "You have three months to live." How would the doctor know? Who is this doctor, a god or something? I find prognoses of death unbelievable, especially when they come from allopathic physicians who are consumed by issues such as gross and cellular pathology, testing (of all kinds), and poisonous medications.

There is a way to see a big picture and it's actually rather easy to understand—that is, after a leading Greek homeopath of our era,

George Vithoulkas, digested it all for us in his book *The Science of Homeopathy*.

Let's consider the human being as a system of overlapping circles that would be diagrammed like a dartboard. If we imagine a human being as three circles of growing diameter, the inner circle would represent the emotional and intellectual level, the second circle would represent the vital organs, and the outer circle would represent the skin and other less-important organs. According to this model, the inner circle is surrounded and protected by the outer circles. This is how it is in real life. Our mental and emotional functions are the most important ones. Without them, we don't exist. In order to provide sufficient housing and energy supplies to these functions, we need vital organs. To create support and protect the vital organs, we need our skin, our skeleton, and all the other devices of our body. When a person is injured, the blood flow is naturally redirected to supply the vital organs first.

I think we can agree that our deepest dimension is the emotional and mental self. Have you ever entered a room and instantly liked or disliked someone there without even talking to him? Think back to college or high school. Perhaps a new professor or student entered the classroom and—in a flash—you just knew you'd get along well. That's how quickly, and deeply, the emotional self works. When we're upset, we cannot function well in any capacity. Emotional pain can be as strong as physical pain or stronger. The mind is important, too. Without clarity of mind, everything else is irrelevant.

Next comes the dimension of the vital organs. We wouldn't be able to feel, think, or do anything if we didn't have a brain or a heart, or a set of lungs, or a liver, and so on. Is this starting to remind you of *The Wizard of Oz*? Remember how important these dimensions were: the Cowardly Lion desperately needed courage (emotion), the Scarecrow needed a brain (vital organ), and the Tin Man wanted a heart (vital organ).

The least important, albeit still valuable, dimension of our being is our skin, bones, and other more surface organs and attributes.

Now when the body aims to heal itself, it tries to express its problems at the most superficial level it can. This fundamental concept in homeopathy relates to the natural tendency of the human body to protect its vital core.

As a child, I went to school with a boy named Michael, who was mentally retarded. He had a large head, but he couldn't read even in the fifth grade. Although this lack of sufficient progress is sadly a reality for many students in America with normal intelligence, it was unheard of in Russia in the 1960s and 1970s, unless a person was developmentally disabled. And Michael was. His behavior was offbeat, too. He often was putting his face close to someone else's, peering into the windows of apartments on the ground floor of buildings, and cursing. Even during the frigid Russian winter, Michael walked around in just shorts and a T-shirt.

To the neighbors, his mother would sometimes say something along these lines: "Michael is not so smart, but at least he's healthy." Wrong!

Michael wasn't healthy. In fact, he was very ill. His most important functions were significantly impaired, although the housing for them (his brain) was pretty large. Please take your time to think about what I tell you next, as it is important. A smart, humorous teenager with terrible pimples is much healthier than a school beauty that sulks around and has suicidal tendencies.

Actor and director Christopher Reeve was one of the most astonishing examples of the accuracy of this three-level diagram of health. After the horseback riding accident that paralyzed him, he lost the use of his body, but he retained his mind and his soul. At the core, he was healthier than thousands of good-looking, but totally dysfunctional, junkies or severely developmentally disabled people, because his emotions and his intellect were intact! I'm not saying he didn't have bad days, as I'm sure he did. But he was resilient. He ultimately died because the structural damage to his body was too severe.

Of course, there are also cases when a physical illness adversely affects a person's emotional and mental state. This means that the person is deeply ill—malfunctioning on all three levels. I've met people with severe cases of cancer who were happy and I've met teenagers with pimples who were almost suicidal. The intimate interplay of various levels of our body and soul creates an opportunity to assess a person's future prospects. A child with severe pneumonia who's happy and surrounded by a loving family has a much better chance of a complete recovery than an unhappy orphan with eczema. In homeopathy, when we look at someone's symptoms, we take the mind-emotions-body into account.

This brings us to the discussion of a slightly different dimension of our health. Obviously, the severity of an illness significantly affects the whole person. Anyone who's had a toothache or a splitting headache will tell you that he felt totally miserable and absolutely couldn't function. I frequently hear statements along the following lines: "I'd rather have my hand amputated than have this terrible toothache" or "There's nothing worse than migraines!" People say such things in the heat of the moment. But how can we properly assess the level of health based on the severity of the illness?

Levels of Health

We can actually distinguish four major levels of health.

Level One Health

I frequently use the example of a young child growing up on a farm to illustrate the ideal state of total health. Generally speaking, children living in a natural environment stay healthy. They wake up in the morning, have a simple nutritious breakfast, and then go out to play. Or they help their parents take care of the family's livestock and pets. The constant contact they have with the environment gives the children's immune systems an opportunity to learn very quickly what is a "friend" and what is a "foe." Every minute of their lives is spent training the immune system. Thus it grows strong and doesn't make mistakes by hysterically overreacting to a harmless thing like cat's dandruff or dog's fur or taking what is a part of the child's body for an enemy. Allergic reactions simply don't exist.

The endocrine system grows strong. They aren't bombarded with junk food and a huge overload of sugar. These children's emotional lives are also simple and healthy.

One day, a Level One child comes home and says, "Mom, I don't feel so good."

The mother checks out his temperature. It's quite high. "OK, son," she says. "Go make some hot tea with honey and get some sleep."

The boy goes to bed and perspires all night. In the morning, he wakes up healthy and ready to go back to school. Aggression (a virus) has been met with immediate strong retaliation (his immune system), followed by a complete elimination of the illness. No emotional or physical consequences of this brief illness are present. Because this boy is healthy, he needs no intervention, no medication. If the cold or the flu were severe, one dose of a homeopathic remedy or herbal medication would probably provide all the help necessary to overcome the illness completely.

Children at this level of health get colds maybe once a year, or even less often. They don't have any allergies or skin problems. They're happy, content, full of energy, and they have pleasant dispositions. I see them on the street, in my friends' homes, or in old movies, but never in my office. They don't need medications. They're completely and independently healthy, and can take care of their daily stresses by themselves.

This is the ideal health we all strive to achieve. Unfortunately, for more children in our stressful and polluted world it seems to be a fairy tale. *But let's not give up!*

Level Two Health

City dwellers and inhabitants of suburban areas are familiar with this level of health, as the so-called civilized environment is terribly polluted. TVs, electronic games, and other sources of loud noise, visual stimulation, and violent imagery contaminate the minds of children. Many chemicals taint the air, water, and food supply. Refined foods have replaced wholesome, more nutritious ones. Drugs have also become a regular part of the culture—and I'm not even referring to illegal street drugs.

God forbid a child has a slight discomfort or a low-grade fever! Medication is introduced right away. Products that should remain hidden deep in the medicine cabinet, to be used only in the state of a *real* emergency, come out prematurely. If children have a scratch, they get an antibiotic ointment. If they have a pimple, they are given antibiotic pills for ten days. For fever, they get aspirin. The vaccination for hepatitis B is now given to infants at two days of age. Why? Just in case something happens.

Are any of these interventions inherently wrong? Of course not! If somebody has a serious wound or a bacterial infection, antibiotics can provide a lot of help. A particular vaccine administered to a population from a high-risk group could be lifesaving. But all of these medications become the enemy of good health when everyone blindly uses them.

The discovery of antibiotics changed the destiny of many severely ill children. Their lives were saved. But then doctors started to prescribe antibiotics for mild and even questionable cases of infections. As a result, new strains of bacteria developed that were resistant to the antibiotics. So we needed new, stronger medications. A vicious cycle was initiated. Hormones (steroids) also saved the lives of many children. Then doctors began prescribing them left and right. Now we're collectively paying the price. Most of our children's immune systems are weak and overstimulated. Their bodies don't know the difference between a friend and a foe. That's Level Two health.

Let's follow an imaginary child named Jessica. Her morning begins with eating cold cereal that contains about a dozen different additives for flavoring, coloring, and preservation, drenched in milk "fortified" with different vitamins. The cows that gave the milk were given hormones every day. Residual hormones have spilt over into the milk. Often Jessica's breakfast is consumed while watching a channel on TV that plays music videos or violent animated programs.

Last night, Jessica sneezed a few times, and her mother gave her an anticongestant "just in case." But this morning, her nose is still stuffed, so Jessica gets a hormonal nose spray. And this is only the beginning of the day! There's more to come. The list of all the overwhelming stressors the child faces could take up a few hundred pages! Jessica's emotions, her immune system, and her endocrine system are overstimulated and weak. She comes home from school feeling under the weather. She has a slight fever. Her mother gives her some aspirin. By the next morning, Jessica is even sicker, so she goes to a pediatrician. The rest of the story is clear: she's ailing for about two weeks.

The majority of relatively healthy children of the modern age belong in the same category as Jessica. They were born with Level One health, but all the numerous stresses put on them by our civilization have made them weaker and dependent on drugs. In a sense, we offer healthy children "crutches" that they don't really need, and their bodies grow up crippled. They don't know how to get by without the immune support.

Level Two children have colds many times a year. These regular colds, flu, and ear infections linger and pile up. So they typically have one or two superficial chronic health problems: conditions such as acne, eczema, ear infections, asthma, attention disorders, or anxiety. But take note! It is important to acknowledge that these children still experience acute illnesses with high fevers. This indicates that their bodies are capable of fighting bacteria and viruses at the superficial levels and coping with everyday stresses.

Children at Level Two have every chance and reason to move to Level One. But reclaiming their health requires breaking the vicious cycle of overmedication. Instead of giving them antibiotics and other medications when they get an acute illness, treatment requires precise homeopathic prescribing and adjustments to their lifestyle and diet. As they still possess resources good enough to shake off all the superficial problems they have, even a single common cold treated with homeopathy can boost their immune defenses to a totally new capacity. Eventually, they'll be able to overcome the adversities of daily life on their own. Like the Level

One farm boy I described, when the immune system is given the chance to fight on its own, it learns and becomes stronger in the process.

Your ultimate goal is to increase the level of your children's health to Level One, or as close to that level as possible. This will make your children *independent* of drugs. You'll learn what you can do as a parent to help your children overcome acute conditions with homeopathy in Part Two. Chronic problems require *constitutional homeopathic treatment*. This approach is described in Part Three.

Level Three Health

Unfortunately, larger numbers of children are moving toward this unsatisfactory level of health. Its main characteristic is the presence of at least one deep-seated chronic illness, such as a severe form of ADHD, depression, autism, asthma, obesity, or an eating disorder. The hallmark of this level of health is a lack of acute diseases. Remember Michael from my childhood? He was seriously developmentally disabled but never had even a simple cold! Obviously, he was not healthy. So what was the reason he didn't catch colds? As his problem was so severe and so central to his being (emotional-mental), the integrative systems of his organism were always on the highest alert possible.

Although the same defensive systems are activated in Level Two children, they don't run at such a high level. They're simply overstimulated and exhausted. In Level Three children, it's a matter of survival. Their bodies continuously attempt to repair what is wrong and fail. The defenses are revved up. A flock of viruses attempting to attack the body hit a firewall of the immune system and burn right away. There's no room for a trivial cold. The battle for survival renders the body unresponsive to more superficial stimuli like cold and flu viruses.

Some parents of children with severe behavioral problems stemming from ADHD or autism have reported that on the rare occasions when their children develop colds with high fevers, their behavior transforms. As one mother said, "For this day or two, my son was 'normal' again." This observation is exciting news to homeopaths. It means that if we learn how to stimulate such children appropriately, we could cure them!

Hahnemann was the first doctor who noticed this phenomenon. He postulated that a stronger acute illness takes over the old, weaker illness. He suggested that if we give a chronically ill person a substance that produces an acute, strong illness, it would cure the chronically ill. It worked. This approach is called homeopathy. Homeopathic remedies are made from substances that in healthy volunteers or victims of accidental poisonings caused symptoms similar to what the patient has. The principle of similars, remember?

Usually, as chronically ill children get better, they start having simple colds. The key then is to treat these acute illnesses either with medicinal herbs or if indicated, with homeopathy. Seek professional guidance on this matter. As treatment goes on, children get stronger and move to Level Two health, and perhaps, eventually, close to Level One.

Level Four Health

This level of health is a sad situation. Most of the Level Four patients that I meet are adults. These individuals have severe, incurable illnesses, such as advanced cancer and long-standing schizophrenia, or they're in the final stages of other fatal illnesses. The goal of treatment is to make them comfortable by alleviating their pain, agitation, and depression. Frequently, a correctly prescribed homeopathic remedy causes a temporary episode of significant improvement. But because the body lacks sufficient resources to support a full recovery, the person reverts back to where he was beforehand. The next prescription may lead to another, less spectacular, improvement, followed by another reversion. Still, it's worth the attempt, as the patient usually feels more comfortable for a while.

Hering's Law: The Direction of Cure

Using information described in the works of Hahnemann, Constantine Hering, one of the founders of American homeopathy, clearly articulated a healing phenomenon that's now known as Hering's Law. This principle states that a homeopathic cure happens from the inside out, from the top of the body moving toward the bottom, and in a chronologically backward sequence. It's as though you were watching a movie of your life in reverse, only faster, but only in terms of symptoms of disease. This natural principle was discovered during the observation of thousands of patients, and through the careful documentation of their chronological development of symptoms as well as of the sequence of their disappearance after homeopathic treatment. Parents may notice it happening when the level of their children's health improves. It's a terrific sign of progress when it occurs.

Many years ago, I prescribed a homeopathic remedy for Boris, a twelve-year-old boy with ADHD and other severe behavioral problems. Over the course of two months or so, Boris stopped hitting other children, he began paying more attention at school, and his teachers reported significant progress to his parents. However, even as Boris continued making strides academically and started having more friends, he also developed asthma. Boris's parents were extremely concerned. At our follow-up appointment, they told me how disappointed they were with the "side effects" of the remedy.

We discussed the case. At first, they didn't grasp that the remedy Boris took more than two months earlier couldn't have been responsible for his asthma attacks because it was so highly diluted and was given only once. Then I asked them if Boris had ever had the same symptoms before. The issue hadn't come up at his initial evaluation. Suddenly both parents said, "Aha!" They told me that when their son was four, he had asthma, which was treated for a few years. Finally, after a course of prednisone, the asthma was gone.

I explained Hering's Law and reassured them that Boris's asthma would probably go away shortly. I also asked if there were any other illnesses they'd forgotten to mention. They recalled that at two Boris had many ear infections and sinus infections that required numerous courses of antibiotics before they went away. They also told me that at twelve months he had severe diaper rash, especially in the front, and later some mild eczema that went away after a few applications of prednisone cream. Their report sounded like a common scenario for children from the late 1980s onward.

These parents were intelligent and realized that all the former issues might return as a result of the homeopathic treatment that Boris received. If so, I assured them that we'd be able to deal with each one successfully without too much pain. All the illnesses they'd mentioned seemed to fit nicely into the picture of the remedy I had given to Boris. Throughout the book, you will see that the *picture of the remedy* must be an exact match with the *picture of the set of symptoms* that it should be used for. Therefore, in this case, all we needed to do was to repeat the remedy when it became necessary.

My prognosis was correct. The asthma was mild and went away rapidly. A few months later, Boris, who was still doing well emotionally, developed an ear infection. It was fairly significant, so I suggested he take a new dose of the same remedy. I know that infection went away, but I don't know what happened after the next year, as Boris was doing well and I lost track of him. Although his eczema didn't come back during the period in which I treated him, if it had, I suspect it would follow a typical healing pattern. I've treated numerous cases of eczema and psoriasis. In general, but not always, the rash initially worsens somewhat. Afterward it clears first on the face, then on the torso and arms, and then it moves finally it clears lower and lower in the body, until it disappears completely.

My eldest daughter's recovery from measles illustrates the direction of cure. First, her cough went away. Then, her rash cleared from her face, trunk, and arms. Finally, it cleared from her legs. The moment the rash cleared from her feet, her fever came down.

In my days of conventional psychiatric practice, I often observed a similar direction of cure. But I'm not always able to persuade my patients that it's a sign of progress or to teach them how to take the opportunity to strengthen their immune system by forgoing interventions. One of my patients was suffering from severe, disabling depression. After completing a course of antidepressants, his depression went away. He then developed a severe bilateral ear infection. With my prompting, he remembered that something similar had happened many years earlier. He'd had a severe ear infection that was treated with antibiotics for a few months. To treat the reemergence of his ear infections, I suggested homeopathy. But he refused. Instead he chose to take a new course of antibiotics. His treatment took a long time. The ear infection subsided, but his mood became significantly worse. Despite my best efforts, it never improved to the extent it had before.

Sadly, we can see clearly that the direction of my psychiatric patient's treatment was wrong. According to the scheme we discussed previously, the cure should have moved from the deepest level (his emotions and mind) to the periphery (in this case, his ears). Using conventional medications, such as antibiotics, suppresses symptoms and drives them underground, neutralizing this healing mechanism. Homeopathy supports the body to express symptoms and thus, essentially, to go back and complete necessary healing.

Unfortunately, there has been no funding available for a retrospective study of the thousands of children who received suppressive treatments for skin problems, like Boris's diaper rash and eczema, to see how deep the pathology goes. No one really knows why a particular child develops a skin disease. We say *predisposition* or *genetics*, but these are only words. Even if we were to identify a particular gene or group of genes responsible for asthma, we don't know what would happen if we altered them—maybe something better or maybe something significantly worse.

The bottom line is that suppressive allopathic treatment of relatively superficial problems doesn't resolve a condition's underlying cause. The body has to deal with it the best it can, and it does so by creating a new set of symptoms, usually on a deeper level. When a child shifts from one level of health to the next with the support of homeopathy, we are likely to see signs of former conditions that have been suppressed reemerging. In children whose immune responses haven't been suppressed with medications, such as my daughters, we see diseases expressed and healed according to the direction of cure. In this way, acute illnesses are not driven underground to take root as chronic illnesses.

Acute Versus Chronic Illness

Today millions of children have chronic illnesses, such as ongoing series of ear infections and sinus infections. In November 2004, I conducted a basic Internet search on the term *chronic disease*. Google turned up 2,180,000 Web pages. Yahoo came up with 611,000. What's the reason that chronic disease is so prevalent in our culture? Why are we facing an increase in disease? Simple. As I've already stated, conventional medicine provides suppressive treatment and transforms acute diseases into chronic ones. We are *all* chronically ill and have been for a long time. But our children in particular are getting weaker. So let me begin to address this concern. Homeopathic theory speaks to this issue. As you'll see later in this book, homeopathy also can provide us with solutions.

Hahnemann was the first physician to classify diseases as acute or chronic. In his main work, *Organon of the Medical Art*, he clearly defined them both. Let's examine his definitions and compare them with definitions embraced by conventional medicine.

Acute Illness

Conventional physicians define acute illness as a condition that starts suddenly and is short-lived. Homeopaths define it as a short-lived condition with symptoms that are different from the usual characteristics of the person and different from the symptoms of any persistent condition the person has.

Acute illnesses have a few important characteristics:

- Their onset is sudden.
- Their progress is rapid.
- They finish their course more or less quickly.
- They have a tendency to heal naturally (that is, without intervention).
- Without treatment, they end in complete recovery or death. (Of course, these days death is an unlikely outcome for an acute illness.)

One of the most obvious examples of an authentic acute illness is an epidemic. Hahnemann actually distinguished individual, sporadic, and epidemic acute diseases. Individual disease doesn't require any explanation. Sporadic disease means a few people in different locations develop an acute illness with the same set of symptoms. During an epidemic, a large proportion of the population suffers from the same disease. If its causative agent (a microorganism) is very strong, the majority of these people will have similar symptoms and may require the same homeopathic remedy.

Symptoms of true acute conditions are usually prominent. If your child has an acute illness, you will be able to see the symptoms. Ideally, you'll also give your child what he or she needs to overcome the illness and remain healthy. In some cases, early symptoms of an illness can be seen only in the first couple of hours. This phenomenon provides parents with a great opportunity to halt the disease in its tracks. I know of many cases when this has happened. This book will teach you how to perform this miracle, using homeopathy, for the great benefit of your children.

Chronic Illness

Conventional physicians define a chronic illness as any disease that develops slowly and lasts a long time. Homeopaths define it as a long-lasting condition, and they emphasize that when it flares up, it may resemble an acute illness. Its symptoms will be the same every time there's an episode, just pronounced.

It's important to note that a chronic illness is not self-limiting. If left untreated or treated allopathically, sooner or later it will get worse.

Before we delve any deeper into these two categories of illness, let's see how important the distinctions between them can be in real life. Imagine that Dr. Watson saw many patients today. Two boys, Sherlock Holmes (who became a great detective in stories by Sir Arthur Conan Doyle) and James Moriarty (who became a brilliant criminal and Holmes's nemesis), left the most remarkable impression. Both had come down with ear infections a week ago and were seen by the doctor immediately. He gave penicillin to each. Today their parents brought them in for follow-up visits. Young Sherlock was cured. He had no pain and showed no signs of inflammation during his ear exam. Clearly, he is a happy, healthy lad.

By way of contrast, James's parents reported that although he had no fever, their son was weak and complained of discomfort in his ear. On examination, there were still signs of inflammation. Dr. Watson had to give James another prescription for a different antibiotic. The poor Moriartys! Their unfortunate son has been having those stubborn ear infections for a few years already.

As you have probably guessed, although their symptoms were similar, Sherlock had an acute ear infection, whereas James actually had an exacerbation of a chronic illness. Sherlock is at Level One of health, as he doesn't have any chronic problems. James is at Level Two of health, as he has a recurring problem. Homeopathic treatment would have been better for the boys than penicillin, because it strengthens all the defense mechanisms of the body. Even with the medication, and perhaps because of similar courses of medication in the past, James has developed chronic *otitis media* (inflammation of the middle ear). So he's probably going to have an ear infection with a similar combination of symptoms every time he's subjected to a significant stressor, like cold weather, an emotional trauma, or a virus.

What could his parents do to help young James regain his health? They need to help him fight his illness all the way through to the end so he can get rid of his current predisposition to ear infections. This requires professional homeopathic help. Imagine what could have happened if James were treated homeopathically the first time he had an acute cold or flu that turned into otitis media. It would be over!

The problem with conventional treatment is that it suppresses the body's symptoms. Although it seems like the illness goes away, in reality the root of the problem is not being addressed. Only individuals who are at Level One of health are cured. But even for them, the unnecessary use of antibiotics is detrimental. Antibiotics always weaken the immune system and in time move a child from Level One health to Level Two health. This is evidenced by more frequent infections and a lower level of energy.

Antibiotics must be used when necessary. Fortunately, in the majority of cases, natural treatment modalities, such as homeopathy, are good enough and antibiotics are unnecessary. Homeopathy helps make children stronger and more independent. Allopathic drugs make patients depend on them more and more by virtue of transforming acute problems into chronic ones.

The majority of children nowadays are at Level Two. They are much more vulnerable to developing chronic problems than earlier generations of children were. Back in his era, Hahnemann noticed some cases in which even the best outcomes of treatment didn't last a long time. He suggested that certain people—now the majority of our population—are predisposed to chronic illnesses from birth. He called this predisposition a *miasm*. Perhaps it's a viable explanation for what's happening to contemporary children.

The Theory of Miasms

Hippocrates was the first physician to use the term *miasm* to describe an infectious agent. The concept has its origins in the Greek word for "taint" or "fault." He postulated that diseases could be transmitted to humans through tainted air and water. After rediscovering the writings of Hippocrates, eighteenth-century physicians adopted the belief that impure airs were responsible for the spread of epidemic diseases. Although Hahnemann agreed that air could carry infectious diseases, he didn't consider the pathogenic material to be gaseous in nature. For instance, he realized that syphilis was a contagious blood disease that could mask itself behind the symptoms of many different illnesses.

Hahnemann redefined Hippocrates' miasmatic approach. After twelve years of thorough clinical observation and historical research, he published a new theory in his book *The Chronic Diseases* in 1828.

According to Hahnemann, all diseases result from inherited predisposition. He insisted that specific morbid tendencies are passed from one generation to the next, and he used the term *miasmatic animalcule* in reference to how they were transmitted. *Animalcule* means "an animal invisible to the naked eye." Dutch naturalist Antonie van Leeuwenhoek invented the microscope and had published his observations of small living animalcules (microbes) before his death in 1723. Hahnemann, although obviously thinking about microorganisms in regard to miasms, didn't know about DNA or genetics. In his book, he offered numerous examples that unequivocally supported his theory.

Originally, Hahnemann identified three major types of miasms. He gave them metaphorical names: the *psoric* (derived from the Greek word *psora*, meaning "itch"), the *sycotic* (derived from the Greek word *syco*, meaning "fig"), and the *syphilitic*. By syphilitic, Hahnemann did not mean the sexually transmitted disease. Although each type of miasm clearly applies to particular diseases, the true essence of the theory of miasms is that people are prone to developing particular sets of problems. Miasms are responsible for diseases of a chronic nature and also lay a foundation for all disease in general. An individual can have any number from one to all three of these major predispositions. Some of the basic characteristics of these three miasms are the following:

- *Psoric.* The entire population shares this predisposition, as it is the most ancient and established a foundation for all other miasms. Its main characteristics are a constant feeling of lack, a need to get more, and a need to be surrounded with more and more protection. This tendency materializes on every level of the human being: anxiety, fears, feeling cold (lack of heat), weakness (lack of strength), conservation, and a constant itch. Children born with a prevalence of psoric features often are plump; cry a lot; have many fears; like to be pampered; like comfort foods, such as milk, eggs, and pastry; need additional layers of clothes; and are prone to frequent itchy skin eruptions.

- *Sycotic.* This miasm represents excess, the need to connect, and the need to spend—a tendency that manifests itself in all the dimensions of the human being, too. Children who possess this miasm tend to be extremely sociable and sexual; love animals; have more energy at night; have physical problems that manifest with excess, such as discharges and skin growths; and feel warm most of the time. As their name suggests, sycotic eruptions resemble little figs. Warts are a good example of these.

- *Syphilitic.* The main characteristic of this miasm is destruction—aimed outwardly and inwardly. It is not a reference to a sexually transmitted disease. I hope none of your children is born with pronounced syphilitic tendencies. These children are prone to behaviors such as torturing animals and teasing or tormenting their siblings. They may also be self-destructive, possibly depressed and even suicidal—sometimes at a very young age. Syphilitic physical problems would include bleeding ulcers and such.

Let me reiterate, microbes do *not* cause the miasms. The theory of miasms is not another, more exotic way of talking about genetics. Many generations ago, microbes and possibly other influences—we don't know exactly what—caused changes in our ancestors. These morbid, or unhealthy, tendencies (miasms) were then passed along to their descendants from one generation to the next. Thus a familial predisposition was created to react to significant stressors *of any kind* in a predictable way.

If an individual with pronounced sycotic tendencies were exposed to gonorrhea, symptoms would flourish quickly in that person. But only a small percentage of people exposed to gonorrhea go on to acquire the miasm. They're either born with it or not. It would take substantial exposure to acquire a new miasm of any kind. Of course, once it did set in, a miasm would be passed on to all succeeding generations.

A common misunderstanding about this theory is to believe that the different miasms are assigned to particular illnesses. In reality, any illness can represent various miasmatic tendencies. It just depends on what stage the illness is in. For example, a person suffering from depression may be uncommonly anxious at the onset of the illness, reflecting a psoric stage. Then the person may become extremely irritable, reflecting a sycotic stage. Finally, if the depression is left untreated, this individual might develop strong suicidal tendencies, which would represent a syphilitic pathology.

Our understanding of miasms has expanded since Hahnemann's day. Currently, homeopaths distinguish as many as ten different miasms. What's important for you to understand, as a parent interested in sustaining your children's well-being, is that the theory of miasms is groundwork for how homeopathy is practiced. It is a partial explanation for why numerous layers of illness may be present in the same individual.

Any time chronically ill children are brought to my office for treatment, I know that their multiple layers of disease probably were created not as much by their miasmatic predispositions as by other modern problems, such as the following:

- Attempts to suppress symptoms of past acute illnesses with allopathic drugs
- Side effects of medications
- Unreasonably aggressive vaccination schedules
- The high level of daily stresses provided by the modern lifestyle

The majority of homeopathic practice is devoted to peeling off multiple layers of illness, if they exist. The ultimate goal is always to restore Level One health. In the next chapter, we'll explore homeopathic remedies, and you'll begin to understand how the principles we've been discussing can very effectively, and easily, be put to use.

Chapter Two

All You Need to Know About Homeopathic Remedies

Remedies are the most important tools of homeopathy. They are the catalysts of healing. Without them, there would be no homeopathy, as the basic principle of our approach is this: like cures like. To produce a powerful effect, however, remedies must be prepared and used according to a strict set of standards. In this chapter, you'll primarily learn how homeopathic remedies are made, as well as how to use them in a safe and efficient way, and a special technique for dosing young children who can't take remedies in pellet form. Before we move on to the specific instructions, let's address a foundational issue: regulation.

How Remedies Are Regulated

Homeopathic remedies have always been at the center of the controversy that surrounds homeopathy. Most M.D.s, and a significant fraction of the general public, have ridiculed the method of using highly diluted substances to promote healing ever since remedies were introduced. Michael Quinn, a well-known and respected American homeopathic pharmacist, writes that "[the methods of homeopathic pharmacy] have been both a blessing and a curse upon homeopathy to this day. [They] are a blessing because they allow us to prepare medicines of great efficacy and low toxicity; they are a curse because a practice of drastically diluting medicines appears so irrational."[1]

Surprisingly, many people think that practitioners make homeopathic remedies themselves. They don't realize that homeopathic pharmaceutical companies in the United States and overseas are monitored for quality and adherence to specific, government-mandated procedures. In the United States, homeopathic remedies are regulated by the Food and Drug Administration (FDA), which recognizes them as legal products.

"Quack busters" frequently accuse homeopaths of sneaking homeopathy into national legislation. Here's the truth. Senator Royal Copeland of New York was chief sponsor of the 1938 Food, Drug, and Cosmetic (FDC) Act that paved the way for the establishment of the modern Food and Drug Administration. To this day, critics of homeopathy still refer to Copeland as the "prominent homeopathic physician," because he was a homeopathic medical doctor and served as president of the AIH in 1908. More interested in administration than in practice, he worked as a dean of New York Homeopathic Medical College from 1908 to 1923 and also as health commissioner for the City of New York from 1918 to 1923. In 1923, he was elected to the U.S. Senate, where he served until his death.

When Copeland introduced the first bill for a complete revision of the obsolete 1906 Food and Drugs Act into the Senate, it launched a five-year legislative battle. The battle turned its course in 1937 after an antibacterial drug called elixir of sulfanilamide, containing a poisonous solvent, killed 107 people, most of whom were children. This event dramatized the need to establish stronger drug safety laws, which until then had been successfully and continually resisted by the drug industry.

The 1938 FDC Act included the following provisions:

- Requiring new drugs to be proven safe before marketing, thereby instituting a new system of drug regulation

- Authorizing standards of identity, quality, and fill-of-container for foods
- Authorizing factory inspections
- Eliminating a requirement to prove intent to defraud in drug-misbranding cases
- Providing that safe tolerance levels would be set for unavoidable poisonous substances
- Adding the legal recourse of court injunctions against violators to the previous penalties of seizures and prosecutions
- Extending regulations to cover cosmetics and therapeutic devices

The FDC Act also recognized the *United States Pharmacopeia* (USP) and the *Homeopathic Pharmacopeia of the United States* (HPUS) as official compendiums. The spirit behind it was to create strict standards for regulating drugs, food, and cosmetics. Both volumes contain definite instructions on how to manufacture medicinal products. We'll explore the homeopathic procedures designated by HPUS later in the chapter.

Senator Copeland did not "sneak" anything into legislation. His homeopathic background helped him to clearly understand the need for strict standards for both homeopathic and allopathic medications and prompted him to take a leadership role in advancing the cause of public safety. As you can see, these very important provisions created a solid foundation for what we now know as the modern FDA.

What's on the Label of a Remedy?

Let's take a look at the label of *Arnica montana,* one of the most commonly used homeopathic medications. It reads as follows:

ARNICA MONTANA 30CH

HPUS

HOMEOPATHIC MEDICINE

ACTIVE INGREDIENT: listed above.

USE: for self-limiting conditions listed below • or as directed by a doctor.

WARNING: Do not use if pellet-dispenser is broken. • **Stop use and talk to a doctor** if symptoms persist for more than 3 days or worsen. • **If pregnant or breast-feeding,** ask a health care professional before use. • **Keep out of reach of children.**

DIRECTIONS (adults/children): At onset of symptoms dissolve 5 pellets in the mouth 3 times a day • or as directed by a doctor.

TRAUMA. BRUISES. MUSCLE SORENESS.

Expiration date: May 2006

New guidelines for homeopathic remedies were established in 1988 and enacted in 1990. According to these rules, homeopathic remedies are divided into two categories: over-the-counter (OTC) and prescription-only. The next point is *very important*. To be classified as OTC, a remedy must be labeled with an indication for the so-called self-limiting conditions it treats. There's a list of forty-five self-limiting categories. For example, the *Arnica* label specifies using for TRAUMA. BRUISES. MUSCLE SORENESS.

The situation resulting from the OTC guidelines can create a lot of confusion in patients' minds. Why? A given homeopathic remedy may have up to a few thousand indications. It's impossible to list them all on the product label. Also, most of the conditions that a remedy cures, problems like depression or asthma, aren't self-limiting. Frequently, a patient buys the remedy from the health food store and is deeply concerned that the indications on the container have nothing to do with the main complaint they have.

Here's an example from my private practice. In the beginning of my career as a homeopath in the United States, I saw an elderly lady with a number of mild neurological problems. The selection of the remedy was not difficult. I clearly saw that I had to prescribe

Causticum, a remedy first introduced by Hahnemann that's made from a mineral. In addition to the other serious systemic conditions that it's used to treat, *Causticum* is also used to treat various neurological conditions. I prescribed the remedy and the lady went to get it. After she read the indication on the label, she became very upset and called me to say how disgusting I was for mocking her. The indication on the label was bed-wetting! Bed-wetting is one of a few thousand symptoms that can be helped with *Causticum*, as well as by many other, much-more-frequently-indicated remedies.

Ever since this awkward incident, I explain to each of my new patients what I just told you. Still I'll frequently get a phone call from a concerned mother, who tells me, "I brought my son for treatment of his migraine and poor attention, and you prescribed a remedy for nasal discharge." And then I explain again that homeopathic remedies are prescribed for the illness in that particular individual, not just for a diagnosis.

Please remember this point when you go to purchase a remedy suggested by your homeopath and also when you shop for remedies on your own. Hundreds of remedies are potentially indicated for particular conditions, depending on the individual characteristics of the intended recipient—your child, you, or another patient. Homeopathy treats people, rather than diseases. Nonetheless regulations require labels to list some conditions.

In accordance with FDA regulations, the label for an OTC remedy has to contain four more pieces of information:

- The concentration of the medication
- Instructions for its use
- Safety warnings
- The expiration date

So far, we already understand a few things. We know the name of the remedy, which is written in Latin. All remedies have Latin names. This makes communication between homeopaths from different countries easy and maintains a clear standard for the sources of the remedies. But what does 30CH after the name of the remedy mean? We know that HPUS indicates that the remedy was manufactured according to the standards of the *Homeopathic Pharmacopeia of the United States*. We also know the use. What about the directions, the warning, and the expiration date?

The Making of a Remedy

In order for homeopathy to be effective medicine, remedies must be highly reliable. The preparation of homeopathic remedies—the way they are manufactured—is done in the same way around the world. The homeopathic pharmacopoeias of various countries vary extremely little from one another, as there's a worldwide standard for each remedy. This includes the description of the raw material that goes into a remedy, the method and time of collection of this material, and the manufacturing process that's responsible for the accurate and consistent preparation of the remedy.

Homeopathic remedies have been prepared in the same manner ever since 1799, the year Hahnemann finalized the process for making them. Currently, twenty-five hundred to three thousand homeopathic remedies are produced from five major sources: minerals, plants, animals, disease tissue (called *nosodes*), and conventional drugs. According to the standards and regulations established by the FDA, a new remedy must be demonstrated to be efficacious in homeopathic practice before it is accepted for inclusion in the HPUS. In other countries, homeopathic remedies are regulated only according to their preparation. Efficacy is frequently disregarded.

The process of the preparation of a remedy consists of a few standard steps, as follows:

- *Step One*. The preparation of what is called the *mother tincture* (denoted by the Greek letter θ). This is a relatively concentrated, alcohol-based solution of the substance.

- *Step Two*. Dilution of the mother tincture in a water-alcohol (ethanol) mixture.

- *Step Three. Potentization*, or activation, of the remedy by *succussion*. Derived from a combination of the German word *schuffeln* and the Italian word *scossone*, both meaning to "shake violently," succussion is a process during which the vial containing the solution is vigorously shaken. Substances that are diluted without being succussed do not share the same healing property as potentized substances.

Steps Two and Three are repeated to achieve a higher *attenuation* (dilution) and greater therapeutic strength. The final product of the process of attenuation is therefore identified as a *specific potency*. For example, you might say, "I am looking for *Arnica montana* in potency 30C (or 6X)." In homeopathy, potency is different than concentration. A preparation containing a higher concentration of source material would actually be of a lower potency than one that's more diluted.

The number with a letter listed on the label informs us about how many steps of attenuation with succussions were performed to achieve a particular potency.

The most frequently used homeopathic potencies are *decimal* (from the Latin word for ten) and *centessimal* (from the Latin word for one hundred). In Latin, numerals are expressed with letters. Ten is represented with an X. One hundred is represented with a C. In some European countries, you may also find decimal dilutions marked with a D (for the Latin word *decimal*).

In the case of centessimal dilutions, as in our *Arnica montana*, the dilution at each step is 1:100. Therefore, by the time the attenuation of 30C is reached, the remedy has been succussed three hundred times and is diluted 10^{60} times.[2]

According to Avogadro's number, a formula used by chemists to calculate the number of molecules in a given amount of any chemical substance, the original substance in a homeopathic remedy disappears at the potency 12C (dilution 10^{24}).[3]

In the case of decimal dilutions, the dilution at each step is 1:10. 12X, for example, means that the remedy was diluted twelve times, succussed 120 times, and the degree of dilution is 10^{12}.

Our *Arnica montana* label reads 30CH. What does the letter H stand for? It means *Hahnemannian*. There are two main methods of homeopathic attenuation: Hahnemannian and Korsakovian. Samuel Hahnemann changed the vial at each step of his attenuation process. By contrast, General Semjon Korsakoff, a Russian homeopath, suggested using the same vial for all the steps. In *Korsakovian* attenuation, every subsequent dilution is achieved by emptying the vial of 99 percent of the previous attenuation, refilling it with fresh solvent, and then repeating the succussion process.

CH indicates centessimal attenuation, Hahnemannian style.

CK indicates centessimal attenuation, Korsakovian style.

Usually, Hahnemannian attenuation is used for the first twelve to two hundred steps in preparing a remedy. Korsakovian method is typically used for higher attenuations.

Preparing Remedies from Insoluble Matter

Hahnemann developed a process that allows us to convert insoluble materials, such as metals like gold or platinum, into a form that can be introduced into the core process just described. This process is called *trituration*.

During this process, the insoluble substance is diluted with nine (or ninety-nine) times its weight of lactose (milk sugar). Trituration used to be performed by processing the mixture by hand using a mortar and pestle. Each step had to be performed for at least an hour. Modern homeopathic facilities now utilize a ball mill instead. This device consists of a cylindrical porcelain jar with a tight lid. The materials are placed in the jar together with very hard porcelain cylinders. The closed jar is then placed on horizontal rollers and rotated by electric motors for approximately two hours at each step.

After two triturations, the resulting remedy, now concentration 3C, goes into the core process. Now operations are part of the usual cycle of homeopathic attenuations.

Extremely High Attenuations

The majority of homeopaths use remedies in centessimal and decimal potencies. Although decimal dilutions do not go higher than 200X, centessimal dilutions can go significantly higher. There are special ways to mark these very high attenuations. 1000C is marked as *1 M* (for the Latin word for 1,000). Consequently, 10M = 10,000C, 50M = 50,000C, CM = 100,000C, and MM = 1,000,000C.

There's another variation that's marked as *LM* (for the Latin word for 50,000). Technically, LM1 = 1:50,000. During the preparation of LM potencies, 1:500 dilution step is added to 1:100 step of the centessimal process. This way, the ratio achieved at each step of the LM dilution is 1:50,000. These dilutions are succussed one hundred times at each step. LM potencies have been becoming more popular in the last ten to fifteen years. The proponents of LM potencies report significantly gentler actions of the remedies.

Making the choice of a particular potency is based on numerous and often complicated factors that should be left up to the professional homeopath. In your own small "family practice," you'll be safe using 30C and in some cases 200C potencies. We'll talk about those in Part Two of this book.

For more details about the different potencies, please read Appendix A.

Pellets, Liquids, Ointments, and Gels

Homeopathic remedies are usually prepared in either pellet or liquid form. The pellets are more popular and generally easier to store and dispense. Their base material is a mixture of sucrose and lactose. They are safe for chemically sensitive individuals and diabetics. Best of all, children love these sweet little pills! The tinctures have an alcohol base and therefore taste slightly bitter.

Pellets are medicated according to a strict protocol. For example, to prepare a pellet form of *Arnica montana* 30C, an 88 percent alcohol solution of the remedy is added to the pellets in a 1 percent ratio. We use 88 percent solutions, because if the concentration of alcohol were to be less than that, the water in the solution would dissolve the sugar pellets. In our case, ten milliliters of the solution of *Arnica montana* 30C is added to a thousand grams of sugar pellets. The pellets are thoroughly shaken to distribute the solution evenly. The pellets are soaked for five minutes and are then dried and packaged. Now the pellets contain *Arnica montana* 30C. Containers with pellets usually hold about eighty pellets of the standard size.

In addition to pellets and liquids, homeopathic remedies are also produced in the forms of ointments, lotions, and gels, which can be applied externally. These have less therapeutic effect than internally consumed remedies. Consumers also can buy homeopathic suppositories and tablets. We'll discuss the administration of these forms of remedies as the book unfolds.

Expiration Dates

Although putting an expiration date on the container is required by FDA regulations, experience shows that homeopathic pellets and tinctures remain active for generations. Remedies made in the time of Hahnemann still exist and are effective. We know that activity of more contemporary products is retained for several decades.

A Little Poison May Cure

The vast majority of parents are unconcerned about the source of homeopathic preparations. They're OK with whatever remedy the doctor chooses. Others become anxious and uncomfortable when they hear names like *Arsenicum*, *Carcinosin*, *Tarentula*, or *Tuberculinum*. The traditional folk names of some of the ingredients in homeopathic remedies don't necessarily sound nice and safe either. Wolfsbane (*Aconitum*), for example, used to be used as a poison on the tips of hunters' arrows. In crude form, it's a strong poison. But a homeopathic preparation of this plant shares fame and popularity in the treatment of acute childhood conditions with *Belladonna*, a homeopathic remedy made from the poison of another powerful plant, deadly nightshade.

How would you feel if a homeopath prescribed your child a remedy made from bushmaster snake venom (*Lachesis*, one of the most popular and effective remedies)? I mean, how does anyone dare offer this stuff to people, let alone children? For years, homeopaths struggled with this issue. Although any homeopath knows how effective and safe homeopathic remedies are, telling parents that their child will be getting a remedy made of wolf spider (*Tarentula*) or cancer cells (*Carcinosin*) has always been difficult.

Conversely, there are remedies made from seemingly inert and harmless substances that in their crude forms couldn't possibly affect anything or anyone for better or for worse, let alone when given in a small dose. For example, the powerful and often prescribed remedy *Natrum muriaticum* is made out of common table salt. One of the cornerstones of constitutional treatment, *Calcarea carbonica*, is made out of oyster shell. Essentially, it is carbonate of lime. *Lycopodium*, a remedy that treats literally thousands of symptoms, is made out of club moss seeds, which are so small that a large amount of them looks like flour. In Hahnemann's day, the seeds were considered biologically inert and were used to cover pills of conventional medications.

Isn't it a total waste of time—even a deception—to offer patients table salt as a cure? And isn't it dangerous to offer patients snake venom or cancer cells? There is a simple way to reconcile the tremendous differences in the materials that go into the making of powerful homeopathic remedies. The key is in the method of preparation. Potentization is responsible for their therapeutic activity. Source materials may be poisons or inert substances. In either case, simple dilutions won't be effective at all. Only serial dilutions accompanied by vigorous shaking at each step do the trick. That's why homeopaths can have it both ways—safe and effective.[4]

There's *no chance* that a homeopathic preparation made out of any substance will carry its infectious or poisonous qualities, because

Hahnemann discovered a perfect method for extracting the curative qualities of various substances. So you can rest assured that your child won't get hurt by homeopathic *Carcinosin* or *Tarentula*.

The majority of classical homeopaths never give prescriptions below 12C, an attenuation at which the active substance in a remedy is exceedingly difficult to detect. The most popular attenuations for these products are 30C and 200C. Essentially, even if a child ate all the pellets in the container at once, poisoning would be impossible.

For thousands of years, humanity has been using poisonous and potentially dangerous substances, in one form or another, for the purpose of healing. Like homeopathy, conventional medicine uses poisonous and biologically active substances. For example, manufacturers have long used whole cells of the pertussis bacteria to produce a vaccine for whooping cough. A new combination vaccine called DTaP (for diphtheria, tetanus, and pertussis) consists of only small, purified pieces of germs. A very old conventional drug, digoxin, is a poison itself if given in large doses; in small doses it helps relieve chronic heart failure. But the same substance could kill if it were taken in its concentrated form. Of course, there are no live bacteria or viruses in any of these preparations. Their difference from homeopathic remedies is that they're significantly less diluted and not potentized at all. Unlike homeopathy, allopathic medicine is not familiar with turning inert substances into medications.

The ancient Romans had a proverb: *"Dosis facit venemon."* Translation: "It is the dose that makes the poison." As far as the safety of a homeopathic remedy is concerned, unnecessary repetition of doses is a much worse issue than the amount of the remedy taken at once. As you'll recall, homeopathic provings are conducted by giving healthy people repeated doses of a substance and monitoring the symptoms they develop.

Of course, a hypersensitive individual might respond poorly to a given remedy. A homeopath would appreciate this fact and make necessary adjustments to accommodate the sensitivity of the patient.

Homeopathic Aggravation

Many parents have heard about the *aggravation*, or "healing crisis," and are concerned that the remedies their children are using could trigger one. What exactly is aggravation? Aggravation is a temporary reaction to the remedy. Usually, it lasts between a few minutes in acute conditions to a few days in chronic conditions. During an aggravation, symptoms of a past illness or of a current acute illness emerge and intensify. This phenomenon is part of the healing process.

Aggravations don't happen all the time, yet an aggravation is usually a clear indication of a correctly prescribed remedy. Symptoms initially worsen and then quickly go away, never to return. In cases when the aggravation is uncomfortably strong, which happens more frequently in constitutional than in acute treatment, the best antidotes are conventional drugs because they work in a manner opposite to homeopathy: suppression.

You don't need to worry about this phenomenon when treating simple acute conditions with remedies in homeopathic concentration 30C. In over twenty years of practice, I can recall only two or three cases when an aggravation was so serious that it required some kind of suppression. All you need to do to prevent aggravations from happening is not repeat the remedy that prompted the aggravation for as long as the symptoms are improving.

There are two populations for whom it is always a good idea to consult professional homeopaths rather than home medicating: pregnant women and infants. In later sections of this book, you'll find possible solutions for a few self-limiting ailments for people in these two groups. To be safe, always consult with your primary care physician to make sure no potentially serious problems are hiding behind a seemingly benign symptom. Appropriately prescribed homeopathic remedies absolutely improve the course of pregnancy and the process of childbirth.

Infants and toddlers tolerate homeopathy perfectly well. The trouble is that they don't speak, and so a layperson might not be able to figure out what remedy is indicated, whereas an experienced homeopath usually can make an accurate determination.

Administration and Storage of Homeopathic Remedies

Modern homeopathic remedies are usually sold packaged in sophisticated, easy-to-use dispensing systems. In administering the pellets, the main principles to follow are not to touch the pills and not to give too many of them to the recipient at the same time. Instructions on the container suggest giving three to five pellets per dose. You are actually welcome to give one or up to ten. Experience has shown that any number of pellets in this range is OK. For the purpose of this handbook, unless otherwise noted, I advise you to take three 30C pellets per single dose. A homeopath usually dispenses one pellet of 30C or a higher potency (for example, 200C, 1M).

Remedies should be taken at least thirty minutes before a meal, and no sooner than thirty minutes after a meal. It is preferable to dissolve pellets under the tongue. But there's evidence that swallowing a homeopathic remedy in this form also works fine.

Some parents prefer giving liquid remedies to their children. Tinctures are widely available. In the case of the administration of the liquid medication, you should give a few drops in a small amount of distilled water. You may also use the *plussing method*, described in the next section of this chapter, to prepare your own liquid dilutions.

Containers holding remedies should be stored in a dry, dark place away from strong odors and electromagnetic radiation. The times that we're living in now present new technological challenges, such as going through an X-ray machine at the airport. A curious homeopath exposed his homeopathic kit to this procedure forty times in a row to determine what kind of impact it would have. His remedies still worked fine afterward. But if you feel concerned, it can't hurt to show your remedies to security personnel and ask permission to bypass the screening. I've never yet met an airport screener who was unfamiliar with homeopathic remedies. (Maybe we should ask them to teach conventional physicians?)

The Plussing Method:
How to Prepare Liquid Remedies

I always tell parents new to homeopathy, "If you thought what you heard so far seemed crazy, wait until I teach you how to dilute remedies."

In cases when you need to administer a remedy in a liquid form, perhaps because a small child is reluctant to swallow a pellet, you can place a pellet in a small (half a liter or less) bottle of spring water. Make sure that you pour out approximately a third of the water from the bottle before adding the pill. Close the lid, wait for five minutes, and then shake the bottle vigorously eight to twelve times by hitting it against a book or the palm of your hand. Then give your child one teaspoon of the water. Close the lid and store the bottle at room temperature. It will remain good for two days. Each time you need to administer another dose, just shake the bottle again and give the child one teaspoon of the water. There's no need to add more pellets.

This method is called *plussing*. It was developed by Hahnemann and is described in paragraph 248 of his main work, *Organon of the Medical Art*. Many homeopaths like plussing and recommend using it for acute conditions, and even some chronic ones. The beauty of plussing is that you increase the potency of the remedy just a little bit each time you perform a succussion. This gives the remedy an additional "kick."

Plussing is useful for cases in which you notice that the initial dose of the remedy did the job effectively, but then the recipient got worse again. That means that the child needs another dose of the same remedy. In such situations, plussing works very well. Repeating so-called dry remedies (meaning just pellets) is OK, too.

I started practicing homeopathy back in the day when there were no plastic bottles of spring water, or at least not in Russia. I used to recommend taking a third of a glass of distilled water, or cooled boiled water; adding a pellet; covering the glass with a saucer; waiting for about five minutes; and then stirring it vigorously for twenty seconds. The results were exactly the same.

This method is reminiscent of Korsakoff's dilution technique. But, of course, if anyone borrowed from someone else's idea, it was Korsakoff using the method proposed by Hahnemann. The following is an example of how the plussing method taken to the extreme of Korsakoff's approach works.

In my days at Columbia University Medical Center, I was friendly with a professor in the field of molecular biology. He was originally from Ukraine, where homeopathy is very popular. One day, he told me about his son having a severe case of acute sore throat. I offered him my services. I went over to his house with a few homeopathic remedies that I'd brought from Russia. Very quickly, I realized that my friend's ten-year-old son, Sammy, was presenting a typical *picture* of *Belladonna*. Remember that the *picture of the remedy* must match the *picture of the set of symptoms* that it is used to treat. His throat was extremely sore, he had a high fever, his pupils were enlarged, and he looked confused.

Because I didn't have many pellets left, I suggested doing the following: they were to perform step one of the plussing method in the glass and give Sammy a teaspoon of the solution. Then they were to pour out all of the water, put in fresh distilled water, stir it, and give the dose again if Sammy began to feel worse. Each time Sammy needed a new dose, the water had to be poured out and new water poured in without adding any more of the remedy.

It worked beautifully. Sammy felt better after the first dose. Then in a few hours, his fever went up, and he was given a teaspoon of water that was added to the glass and stirred after the original solution was poured out. After the second dose, the effect lasted even longer. The procedure had to be repeated only one more time.

Since then, I've prescribed homeopathy for practically all the members of the professor's family, including some grandchildren and a great-grandmother, with great success. I'm not asking you to go to such an extreme, but certainly the plussing method has its place in homeopathy.

Is It OK to Combine Remedies with Conventional Drugs?

There's an old joke that reminds me of how many people feel about homeopathy and conventional medicine. It goes something like this: a man gets stranded on an island. Fifteen years later, a cruise ship rescues him. Before leaving the island, the man offers the captain a tour. The captain is surprised to see two large huts standing opposite each other. The man explains, "This one is the shrine I go to, and that one is the shrine I *don't* go to."

Although a few people in our culture use homeopathy or conventional medicine exclusively, in reality the majority of people combine them. If homeopathy or allopathic medicine is the "shrine" your family generally visits, and now you're considering visiting the other one, you need to be able to answer one of the following questions before your child receives treatment:

- "If my child is taking conventional drugs, can I give him or her homeopathy?"
- "If my child is taking homeopathy, can I give him/her conventional drugs?"

The safety of your child is obviously the main objective of any treatment strategy. Everything else comes second. But let's put one idea on the table from the beginning of this discussion. For better or worse, allopathic physicians provide more than 90 percent of the medical assistance that people receive in the modern, so-called civilized world. But M.D.s know extremely little about homeopathy. Their personal attitudes influence your care.

You, as a parent, wish to give your children the best holistic care possible, and possibly you're upset that your physician doesn't know about homeopathy. If so, what can you do? Should you stop seeing the conventional doctor? No. But if and when there's a window of opportunity for you to try a homeopathic solution, I suggest

that you seize it. You can always fall back on conventional medicine. A rational combination of the two medical approaches would
be ideal for pediatric, as well as adult, health care.

Millions of children are alive today due to the existence of sterile surgical techniques, blood tests, magnetic resonance imaging,
and rationally used antibiotics. The list of allopathic medicine's
tremendous gifts is long. But in an ideal world, whenever there was
a need, we'd first apply homeopathy, trying to resolve both acute
and chronic conditions by strengthening children's natural defense
mechanisms. On occasion, we'd also turn to surgery. The use of
heroic allopathic measures, including antibiotics, would be reserved
only for those patients whose defense mechanisms couldn't overcome their illnesses without outside help, situations when the measures were absolutely warranted.

In this ideal world, homeopaths and allopaths would work
together for the good of humanity. The ultimate outcome would be
a much stronger, healthier generation of children, who would suffer fewer chronic illnesses, experience less mental illness, and
engage in less crime. Unfortunately, this kind of teamwork rarely
exists today. Because the ideal is still a dream, how do you navigate
the course to your children's total health?

Four Guidelines for Coordinating
Your Child's Health Care

It's important to find a doctor who'll be able to coordinate the various treatment modalities as they play out together, a health care
"quarterback." Locating such a person may not be an easy task. It is
much easier in major cities, where there are usually integrative
health care centers in which conventional providers who are
CAM-friendly work hand in hand with homeopaths, acupunctur-
ists, and other types of alternative practitioners. (CAM is the term
for complementary and alternative medicine.) If you cannot find a
place like that, the next best option is to ask if your pediatrician or
family physician is open to CAM. Even better, seek a primary care
physician who practices homeopathy.

Unfortunately, you may wind up feeling that you need to handle the coordination of treatment on your own. In that case, here are four guidelines you need to follow:

• *Guideline One*. Regardless of how incorrect and potentially damaging you believe the current treatment regimen of your child is, *please do not discontinue conventional medications without professional medical advice*. You need to be clear on this point. A sudden cessation of medications may put a significant stress on your child's system—one so significant, in fact, that your child's condition may become much worse than before.

I cannot begin to tell you how often homeopaths have to face the following dilemma. The parents have "tried everything" and have come to the homeopath as a last resort, hoping for a miracle. Now they immediately want all the medications stopped, either because the drugs aren't working or because there are side effects. Even as I was writing this chapter, I had to deal with a situation where a couple were so excited by the improvement they saw after their son took a homeopathic remedy that they suddenly took him off his prescription drugs. Predictably, their son wound up getting sicker and they panicked.

Please understand that the only objective that professional homeopaths have is to improve your children's health. And we need to do it in a safe way. If we rush the situation, your child, who is already weak, may experience more damage.

The danger of suddenly discontinuing medication exists whether or not you subsequently give your child homeopathy.

• *Guideline Two*. Do not begin homeopathic treatment and allopathic treatment at the same time. With rare exceptions, you should use only one of these modalities at a time. If your child has chronic ear infections, for example, and currently is showing all the signs of a severe infection, it's a good idea to let your child undergo a full course of antibiotics first, and then go see a homeopath. The homeopath can help you cure the chronic problem that is causing repeated ear infections. Combining antibiotics with homeopathy wouldn't make sense, as these two approaches work in opposite directions. The former suppresses symptoms to achieve relief, whereas the latter helps express symptoms in order to cure them. In addition, if changes *do* occur while you're using both approaches simultaneously, you won't know to what to attribute them.

Of course, it's always your decision which way to go. For another condition, you might decide to ask a homeopath to treat your child first, before trying a conventional medication. The important part is not to procrastinate in making a decision, because a delay may allow illness to progress to a dangerous level. The same holds true for any condition in which you have to face a choice between homeopathic or allopathic treatment. Be proactive.

Good news. In acute situations, correctly prescribed homeopathic remedies work swiftly—usually right away. Therefore you won't be in doubt for long about the results of your decision. But in some cases, it can take a few tries to narrow in on the right remedy, the simillimum. So please don't wait until the very last moment! I often hear statements like this one. (The conversation happened at the end of July.) "Doc, we waited for so long and finally decided to start our son on Ritalin. Now we absolutely have to get results by the end of August, so you have three weeks to try." An impossible proposition!

Make up your mind if you want to use homeopathy, then determine your window of opportunity, and if it's too short at the moment, use whatever conventional method you need to in the meantime, and then bring your child to the homeopath at the beginning of the next window of opportunity. Or if there isn't an opportunity, do what's suggested in Guideline Three.

• *Guideline Three.* If your child has already been taking conventional medication for a few months, homeopathic treatment may safely be added. Your child's major defense mechanisms will have already adapted to the combination of stresses caused by the illness and the medication.

As I indicated in Guideline One, your child needs to keep taking the conventional medications. Finding the right remedy for a child who's been receiving suppressive allopathic medications is difficult. But as homeopathy begins to work, the improvement will be obvious to the allopathic physician, and then discontinuation of the medication is possible. More and more allopathic physicians accept the fact that a large number of children receive help from CAM providers. Professional dialogues are developing.

• *Guideline Four.* If your child is receiving homeopathic treatment, all new symptoms and conditions should be managed with the participation of your attending homeopath. Symptoms may only be evidence of a brief healing crisis, which from a homeopath's perspective shows the healing process is on track.

Before you do anything else—even apply a cream, give an aspirin, or use an inhaler—contact your homeopath—*right away*. Jumping the gun and rushing into a course of suppressive treatment can severely disrupt homeopathic treatment. We don't want to interfere with nature. I'll give you an example of what can happen.

A few years ago, I treated Linda, a beautiful ten-month-old angel. Almost since her birth, Linda had an ear infection that was treated with numerous courses of antibiotics. She went on to develop severe asthma attacks that required frequent visits to the ER. As her pediatrician knew about homeopathy, he suggested that her parents see whether or not I could help. The parents called to make an appointment while Linda was finishing a course of prednisone. We met a week after this hormone therapy was finished.

Linda's illness was severe and had frequent exacerbations, but she was a happy, personable child. Her emotional level was intact. Put together, these signs indicated that she was fighting her illness. For all the purposes of my evaluation, Linda was clearly at Level Two health. Her symptoms and family history made the choice of remedy obvious. After taking only one dose, Linda began to improve and was illness-free in a few short weeks. The pediatrician was comfortable with the results. Linda didn't need further treatment.

At Linda's six-week follow-up, I reinforced the same rules we're talking about here. Parents in my practice are told everything that you're reading. Nonetheless, a few months later, I received a phone call early in the morning from Linda's mother, who was frantic. The night before, her daughter had developed a fever of 101.3, so Mom decided to give her some Tylenol. Although the fever went down due to the drug's suppressive action, in the morning Linda developed a cough and started to wheeze. Mom was extremely alarmed that Linda was having an asthma attack.

Because her daughter was suffering that day, I recommended to Linda's mother that she give Linda an asthma medication inhaler. By then, there really was no other choice but to resort to a conventional drug. I told her to take Linda to see her pediatrician ASAP, and then afterward to come see me. I immediately phoned the physician, who also reached out to Linda's mother to ensure that in her state of panic she wouldn't forget to come see him that morning and receive additional instructions, if necessary. It is my belief, however, that the entire asthmatic episode might have been avoided if Linda's fever had been allowed to run its course with only a little help from homeopathy.

Of course, you should be prepared to go to the emergency room if the acute problem is severe enough to warrant it. Go to the ER if you can't get in touch with your homeopath in the course of ten to fifteen minutes. But if your child has only a mild fever of 100.1 degrees and is active and happy, you could wait a little bit longer. Use common sense. When in doubt, always seek help.

Is It OK to Combine Remedies with Other Forms of Alternative Medicine?

As indicated previously, it's better not to use more than one health care modality at a time, even when the treatments are natural, or biologically based, such as herbs and plant extracts. Theoretically, there's no valid distinction between the same person taking numerous conventional medications and taking numerous alternative medications, or any other combination of conventional and alternative product. It is always polypharmacy, which confuses the body's responses because different medications send different, sometimes opposite, messages to the body.

What about giving a child an additional homeopathic remedy (or more) while that child is being treated by a homeopath for a chronic problem? What harm can come from that? It is the same thing! *Polypharmacy*.

A good description of what can happen when various treatments are combined is contained in the following fable. A fool hires a lobster, a stork, and a donkey to move a carriage. He thinks the job will get done faster this way. The lobster will pull on the carriage from the river; the stork will pull from the sky; and the donkey from the ground. After hours of effort, however, the carriage doesn't move an inch. Why? Where does the fool's plan go awry? The laborers are pulling in opposite directions. Similarly, when several medications are taken, the body's functions work in opposition.

By the way, this principle of not mixing different forms of treatment can even be true for CAM modalities, such as osteopathy and craniosacral therapy, that don't involve the consumption of substances. I'll explain why a bit later in the chapter.

Most parents feel compelled to do the best they can for their children. Many assume more is better. Today children often have busy schedules: a soccer game Sunday morning, ballet class Sunday afternoon, martial arts Monday and Thursday, cheerleading practice Tuesday, piano and violin lessons on alternating Wednesdays, spinning class Friday night, and Japanese calligraphy Saturday. How's that for a happy childhood?

I've met many children whose parents regularly take them to see practitioners of Chinese medicine, Ayurveda, craniosacral therapy, osteopathy, and so on. The schedule offered by many so-called holistic specialists is similarly hectic. Their aim is to "chelate heavy metals" or "boost the immune system." Such children get caught up in a vicious cycle of being overtreated and overprescribed alternative medicines. Yet they don't get better. The popular premise called *synergism*, the concept that dissimilar modalities applied together are mutually supporting, is obviously wrong. More is *not* better.

Recently, the parents of two autistic children who are my patients underwent a highly educational experience. For years they'd combined a variety of CAM approaches. After homeopathic treatment, the children improved somewhat, but not to a spectacular extent. Then, due to financial difficulties, the parents had to stop bringing them to all the care providers except for the homeopath. Surprisingly, the children started to improve at a much faster rate. This aptly illustrates my point: each CAM modality can bring about significant improvement. Still it's better to utilize them judiciously, not necessarily at once.

By the way, many of the children I meet have never had milk, bread, or candy. In fact, there's no real food in their lives anymore. Instead their meals contain "proteins," "fats," "carbohydrates," and "supplements." Sounds like a nightmare already? It is!

Why don't we stop and think about nutrition for a second. If children have Level One health, they don't need vitamin and mineral supplements, and they don't have to avoid eating regular foodstuffs. Yes, your children need to eat a balanced diet. Certainly, buying organic produce and products is a good idea, if you can afford them. Eating organic prevents chemicals and hormones from being introduced into children's bodies. But only children with compromised health need to make *temporary* adjustments in their diets, such as eliminating wheat or dairy to control their allergic responses.

What about children with acute illnesses? Isn't it better to hit the immune system with a powerful booster, such as an herb? Actually, it isn't necessary for children with Level One health. They only need gentle "reminders" of what their bodies naturally know to do. A homeopathic remedy is fine for this purpose.

Children with Level Two and Level Three health do remarkably well on homeopathic treatments when they are faced with acute ailments. Of course, some parents feel the need to introduce herbs into the mix at these times, and this is fine—especially when someone doesn't really know what remarkable results can be achieved by using homeopathy. Perhaps they've just read about it. While you're learning about homeopathy, try to use as few herbal supplements as you possibly can. Less is more with any treatment approach.

I was pleasantly surprised to learn that cranial therapists and osteopathic physicians ask their patients not to combine other CAM modalities with what they're doing. I've had personal experiences with Ayurvedic, Tibetan, and Chinese physicians, and most of them also suggest not combining modalities. There are two main reasons. First, we don't really know how various modalities interact with one another. All of them, including homeopathy, are built on the belief that illness and cure happen on an energetic plane. The influence that each of these modalities has on the human energy system is very subtle. If there is a chance that they'll interfere with one another, the consequences are unpredictable.

Second, if we combine modalities, how can we understand what did or didn't work or what caused harm if the condition worsens? Allopathic medicine works on a concrete, physical level. That's why homeopathy may be superimposed on allopathic drugs without causing the kind of problems just described for CAM modalities.

Children don't need to go at the same time to every single health professional that parents can find. But if your child is suffering from a chronic illness for which you are seeking homeopathic treatment, you should make an informed decision of what other therapies are absolutely necessary to keep doing—steps such as continuing a regimen of herbal medications the child is already on—and what steps can wait.

If your child has been on the same CAM treatment regimen for a few months and you decide to see whether homeopathy can make a positive difference, adding a remedy to an already established therapy presents less of a problem than it would otherwise. Your child's body has probably stabilized its functions by now.

Of course, there are exceptions.

It is not uncommon for children receiving treatment for chronic conditions to develop acute ailments, such as colds and flu. In fact, acute illnesses that occur during ongoing constitutional treatment can be signs that your child's overall level of health is improving. But how should you handle an acute illness? Can you give your child a homeopathic remedy, or would that nullify the ongoing treatment? Can you use herbs? The best thing to do is to consult with your treating homeopath.

If the illness is a true acute illness, meaning that your child has developed new, uncharacteristic symptoms in the midst of an ongoing illness, taking a new homeopathic remedy may or may not be indicated. Speak to your homeopath about it to be certain.

The rule of thumb is that herbal supplements are safe in such instances. They don't suppress the body's innate healing processes, nor do they interfere with homeopathy. Like herbs, Bach remedies are safe to use, as these formulas are made from flowers. Aromatherapy oils are very safe, so long as they're not ingested. Just be careful using eucalyptus, clove, mint, and peppermint oils around a child who is receiving homeopathic treatment. These oils may antidote, or nullify, the effect of homeopathy.

There's a potential complication, too. Symptoms that seem to be acute might actually be a part of the healing process initiated by homeopathy. According to Hering's Law, if your child has ever had a similar *symptom picture* (as discussed previously, this is a particular group of symptoms) in the past, those symptoms may now be reemerging. If so, the situation becomes more complicated. Your homeopath *must* be involved in the decision-making process.

This leads us to the next chapter, "Developing a Partnership with Your Homeopath."

Chapter Three

Developing a Partnership
with Your Homeopath

So far, you've learned the basic principles of homeopathic theory and general instructions for using homeopathic remedies. Topics covered in this chapter include preparing for a professional homeopathic evaluation, understanding how practitioners determine the right remedy, the pros and cons of doing Internet research as a layperson, and a comment on when conventional medicine may be a better choice for your child than homeopathy. We'll answer the questions that parents ask most frequently. Please remember, you can never make a misstep by soliciting the advice of a homeopath.

In future chapters, we'll explore the process of selecting remedies on your own for many common acute conditions. A homeopath can counsel you. We'll also tackle specific chronic conditions—mental, emotional, and physical—that must be treated constitutionally. These are complex scenarios that require support from a properly trained homeopath. By helping you understand what to expect and how homeopaths work, we hope that the ideas presented here will help your interactions run smoothly.

How to Prepare for Professional
Homeopathic Evaluation

When they first come to see a homeopath, thoughtful parents often bring copies of tests that have been done by conventional physicians and then spend a good portion of the consultation describing step-by-step what other nonhomeopathic physicians and CAM practitioners have said and done. Even though this kind of information is certainly important and useful, it shouldn't become the main thrust of a homeopathic evaluation.

Minute details about someone's condition help homeopaths characterize that person as a unique individual. In keeping with the context of their practice, conventional doctors need people to be the same as one another. They use test results—details—to classify people into groups.

Homeopaths need to know what's going on or *not* going on, on the pathological level. But it would make more sense for you to create a synopsis of any earlier findings about your child's condition and present it briefly. Bring conventional test results with you, so the homeopath can look at them.

Don't bother going into much detail about what a Chinese medicine or Ayurvedic medicine specialist said. These popular alternative forms of medicine have theories and terminology that don't cross over into homeopathy. They can be effective; nonetheless we cannot utilize their databases for homeopathic prescribing.

The primary thing a homeopath needs to figure out during an evaluation is what makes your child different from all other children experiencing the same problem. Characteristics that make your child different from everyone else could include the exact location of the condition, the time of day or night when it's better or worse, and what kind of natural things you do that improve or complicate the problem.

Homeopaths also need to know what has changed since your child initially developed the problem. They are interested in your child's temperament, what kinds of fears your child has, how and in what positions your child sleeps, and what kinds of food your child craves or refuses. Seemingly strange questions like, "Does he bite his nails?" or "Does she uncover herself in her sleep?" often provide a lot of useful information.

A homeopath needs to be able to understand what changes were brought about by the illness and how your child interacts with the outside world. Is she shy or very outgoing, is she very responsible and organized, or is she kind of sloppy? Usually, parents have no difficulties answering these sorts of questions.

You'll have an even better idea of what your homeopath needs to know if you try to find remedies for acute problems or just flip through Part Two of this book.

What Tools Do Professional Homeopaths Use to Find the Correct Remedy?

The main tools of homeopathy are observation and interview. A child can sometimes respond to the clues contained in direct questions. But subtle signs and symptoms that the homeopath gathers as a result of observation and indirect questioning are very important. Information provided by direct observation is graded higher than any other. It gives the best insight into what's going on. The skill of clinical observation and gathering relevant, frequently subtle information is critical. It is developed through experience and dedication. No technical device or book can provide these skills.

The ability to notice subtle clues is certainly defined by the personality and intellectual characteristics of the health care provider. In my opinion, this requirement alone creates a significant barrier to homeopathy for a large number of conventional physicians. It's truly difficult for most of them to appreciate how important this type of information is. For example, an allopathic physician is going to treat a right-sided ear infection in the same way as a left-sided ear infection. The treatment? An antibiotic. The reason? The database this physician uses doesn't appreciate the variation. There's no antibiotic specific to a particular side of the body. "What a ridiculous thought!"

For a homeopath, such information is considered significant, however. Different people have different strengths and weaknesses. Everyone knows that. Unfortunately, frequent use of suppressive treatment shuts down the attempt of the body to show us what is wrong. Certainly, it would be nice to have a simple laboratory test that indicates what remedy to give, but it doesn't exist. No single test can describe the complexity of a particular human being with a unique set of symptoms. Many different tests are still disconnected from one another and do not unite in a cohesive pattern that would be characteristic of a particular remedy.

After the data are collected, the homeopath needs to process them in a meaningful way to appreciate the whole picture of the presenting problem. As discussed in previous chapters, this picture has to be matched perfectly to the picture of a remedy. Only a completely identical match is the one remedy that's indicated for a particular person with a particular problem or set of problems—in homeopathic parlance, this remedy is called a *simillimum* (meaning "similar" in Latin). A simillimum produces a cure.

Finding the simillimum for an acute problem in an otherwise healthy child is relatively easy, because the child's body speaks to us in a clear language of prominent characteristic symptoms. That's why you'll be able to use homeopathy to treat most acute ailments in your own children. In complicated situations, finding the simillimum could be more difficult. Then you'll need professional homeopathic guidance.

The *Materia Medica*

Each patient has many symptoms, and each remedy treats thousands of symptoms. How do we ever find an exact match? Anything short of that will provide less than complete cure.

Early homeopaths were able to hold all of the symptoms of a few dozen remedies in their heads. But soon, two main reference tools were developed. The first one is the *Materia Medica*. An adequate translation from Latin for this would be the "homeopathic pharmacology." Hahnemann wrote the first two-volume work of this kind. Called the *Materia Medica Pura*, it was published from 1811–1821. Then, in 1828, Hahnemann published *Chronic Diseases*, a book that contained detailed descriptions of additional homeopathic remedies. During his lifetime, Hahnemann reported the results of provings and clinical observations for about a hundred remedies. Information provided in these two books remains some of the most reliable in homeopathic literature.

Later authors, including Constantine Hering, wrote new volumes of *Materia Medica* with more remedies described. In the spirit of the old tradition, modern books on homeopathic pharmacology are still called *Materia Medica*. These volumes now contain thousands of pages of detailed information on every symptom that was either described during a proving or cured in many patients by a particular remedy. The *Materia Medica* lists these symptoms so they can be matched with the symptoms in the patient.

All *Materia Medica* present their information on a given remedy in the same order. Each description begins with the origin of the remedy and general characteristics of the effects it produces. Then the description goes system by system. The first category is always *mind*, meaning what mental effects fit the picture. The last category is *modalities*, meaning what makes the symptoms better or worse and when do the symptoms appear or disappear. Next there's a list of conditions that usually respond to the remedy. Then there's a list of remedies that are similar as well as their differences. Finally, there's a list of antidotes, other remedies that would counteract this remedy's action.

Some remedies cure literally thousands of symptoms (see a sample in Appendix A). For example, the entry for *Calcarea carbonica* contains over eight thousand symptoms! I've actually met people able to remember almost all of the symptoms for a few frequently prescribed major remedies, such as that one. A good homeopath can remember the characteristics of a few hundred remedies. But not of all of them! Today several thousand remedies have been characterized.

The *Repertory*

The second book that homeopaths turn to is called the *Repertory* (derived from the Latin word *repertus*, meaning "to find"). It's a cross-reference tool that lists all remedies known to be associated with a particular symptom.

In 1805, Hahnemann created the first handwritten *Repertory*. It has never been published. Another handwritten *Repertory* was created by one of Hahnemann's close students, George Jahr. The most famous ones were drafted by Clemens Maria Franz Von Boenninghausen (1832) and James Tyler Kent (1877) (see Appendix C).

Born in the Netherlands in 1785, Boenninghausen became the brightest star of the homeopathic constellation, second only to Hahnemann. Early in his life, he rose to prominence as a lawyer and held the position of king's auditor, which was comparable to being attorney general. He resigned this position in 1810, returned to his estate, and studied agriculture. Shortly after that, he became president of the Court of Justice for the newly recognized Prussian provinces of Rhineland and Westphalia. He excelled in this position, too. Then in 1827, at age forty-two, Boenninghausen contracted tuberculosis (TB) and the course of his life changed direction.

Remember, this occurred more than a hundred years before the discovery of antibiotics. There was no hope for a recovery. Boenninghausen prepared to die. In a farewell letter to one of his friends, Dr. Weihe, who was a botanist, he asked for advice. But unknown to Boenninghausen, Weihe had studied with Hahnemann. After learning details about his friend's condition, Weihe mailed him a homeopathic remedy. In a few months, Boenninghausen was 100 percent cured of TB!

The light went on. From then on, Boenninghausen dedicated all of his time to studying homeopathy. Soon he became one of the most prominent theoreticians and writers in the field. A layperson, he was granted permission to practice homeopathy in 1843. Consequently, Boenninghausen came to be highly recognized for creating the first homeopathic *Repertory*, one of the main tools used to find a correct remedy.

James Kent's *Repertory* remains the most admired. Its structure, or the way it presents information, as well as the information it contains, have been used as the backbone for all subsequent repertories. The descriptive way to write a symptom in the *Repertory* is called a *rubric* (which refers to a category).

Rubrics are organized according to a scheme first introduced by Kent. The first, and one of the largest, sections is mind. The last, and also a very large section, is *generalities*. This lists symptoms that indicate the relationship of the person to the outside world. These two sections are considered to be the most important. The rest of the *Repertory* is divided anatomically and according to various systems of the body. (See a sample page from the *Repertory* in Appendix C.)

Remedies within each rubric are listed in alphabetical order and graded on a scale from four to one. So when a remedy has a particular characteristic in a remarkably strong way, it is assigned a four, and its name is printed in **bold, <u>underlined</u>** letters.

A remedy with clear, strong, and common indications for this particular rubric is graded as a three. Its name is printed in **bold** letters.

A remedy whose use for a particular rubric is less clear and strong, although it is supported by clinical results, is designated as a two. Its name is printed in *italics*.

Finally, a remedy with infrequent and weaker use for this particular rubric is designated as a one. Its name is printed in regular type.

By cross-referencing important symptoms, homeopaths arrive at a few possible choices of a remedy for their patients. They then make a final decision, using their clinical experience. Usually, the final decision-making process involves studying the *Materia Medica* of a few remedies. Homeopaths work with these books all the time. The most popular contemporary repertories are entitled the *Synthesis Repertory* and the *Complete Repertory*.

With the advent of computers, the *Repertories* and *Materia Medica* have become part of sophisticated homeopathic software. Modern computer programs make searching for the right remedy much easier. Nonetheless a well-trained homeopath still remains the core component of the prescribing process.

Some parents have told me that they purchased expensive homeopathic software for their home computers only to discover that every search ended with the remedy *Sulphur*, a remedy represented in the majority of rubrics. That's why parents really cannot circumvent the expertise of a professional homeopath if they want to provide adequate care for a chronically ill child.

Doing or Not Doing Internet Research

Should you do or not do Internet research? My short, simple answer is this: don't do it until you've finished reading Part One of this book. These four chapters will give you enough background to be able to navigate though an enormous amount of information and—most important—misinformation that you are likely to find on the Internet.

One of the main features distinguishing online material from the material in published books, such as this one, is that anyone can post any statements they want online, because there aren't any checks and balances in place. In contrast, not only was this book written by a board-certified homeopath, but the company that published it authenticated my credentials. In addition, the board of trustees of the AIH approved me as the author. Finally, before the book went into print, the manuscript was read and fact checked by a number of experts. Nothing comparable happens on the Internet.

I did a lot of research, including Internet research, during the process of writing this book. I can't even begin to tell you how many ridiculous things about homeopathy are out there. But I know homeopathy, both its theory and practice. I can tell the difference between accurate and false statements. Laypersons frequently can't.

Many consumers of homeopathy are tempted to read about various homeopathic remedies. This creates an enormous problem. Most of the commonly used homeopathic remedies are capable of treating hundreds, often thousands, of symptoms. One really needs to understand these remedies very well in order to make sense out of the various descriptions readily available on the Internet.

Psychologically based descriptions are especially popular. Easy to read, they create a false sense of deep understanding of the remedy. But what do you do if someone just has a fever? How deep do you need to go? And if you do need to go deep into your child's psyche, are you trained to do so? What position should you take on homeopathic vaccination and prophylaxis?

All of these and many other questions are answered in this book. After reading the book carefully, you probably won't need much of the Internet "research," but if you are still curious, you might decide to investigate anyway.

At that point, you'll be safe, because you'll be more knowledgeable about the important principles of homeopathy. You'll be grounded with roots growing directly from the brain of Samuel Hahnemann.

Just remember, at every single homeopathic conference I've attended, the most popular topic was the *Materia Medica*. It is also one of the most useless topics. The real main issue that parents need to understand is homeopathic theory. This enables you to successfully treat your children's acute ailments on your own and to be able to navigate the path of their constitutional treatment under the guidance of a homeopath.

What Is Constitutional Treatment?

Identifying the correct remedy for a chronic condition is a different and more complicated process then finding a remedy for an acute ailment. To find any remedy, homeopaths need to know what changes—characteristic to this particular person—have been caused by a particular illness. In acute conditions, changes usually are obvious because they are new and strong. The integrative systems of our bodies try to externalize problems to protect the most important vital organs and systems. Symptoms are easy to recognize, and a relatively limited number of remedies tend to be useful.

Cocculus and *Tabacum* are most frequently indicated for the treatment of car sickness. The majority of people will exhibit signs and symptoms of these remedies, and only a smaller population will require alternatives. Similarly, the majority of the population will respond very well to either *Apis* or *Ledum* when stung by an insect, and only a smaller group will exhibit signs and symptoms of a few other remedies.

We can also look at the situation from the deeper perspective of homeopathic philosophy and say that a person who has responded to stress with certain signs and symptoms in one event, most probably will have a similar systemic response to any severe stressor. These stressors could be of an emotional nature (for example, a natural disaster, a terrorist attack) or a physical nature (for example, a severe infection, a severe trauma, surgery, having a baby). A stress is still a stress. The symptoms might be panicky: severe fear with a feeling of imminent death, accompanied by restlessness, heat, an expression of extreme fear on the face, and an unquenchable thirst for cold drinks.

A relatively healthy individual has a limited repertoire of symptoms that develop in response to various types and degrees of acute stressors. So a particular "melody" from this repertoire is played depending on what demand is being placed on the person at a particular time. Different people have different repertoires. That's why two people exposed to the same stressful event—for example, an earthquake—react in two ways. Let's say one goes into an *Aconitum* state (characterized by extreme agitation and panic), another into a *Gelsemium* state (characterized by extreme weakness and paralyzing anxiety).

If left untreated, these two individuals may either recover on their own without any trace of problems, or they may go into a deeper pathological state with more and more symptoms created on the emotional and physical levels. Diseased states have a tendency only to get worse, with pathology going deeper and deeper.

The reality of our era is that by the time a sick person meets a homeopath, a number of other health professionals were already involved in that individual's treatment. A number of opportunities to address the problem when it was still relatively superficial were missed. The past use of suppressive methods of treatment makes the deciphering of the code of the illness even more difficult. It also alters and complicates the mechanisms used by the person's body for its healing response. Layers and layers of issues with their own patterns of response to various stressors have been superimposed on whatever remaining original, healthy, self-regulating mechanisms there are.

Because the person is now chronically ill, the changes the homeopath must identify can be extremely subtle, and the process of choosing the right remedy is laborious. Even in cases when a very well-known remedy is indicated, symptoms may not be as clear and straightforward as we might hope. The process of finding the correct remedy in these situations requires a deep understanding of the main principles of homeopathy, combined with clinical experience and detailed knowledge of homeopathic pharmacology. In this type of prescribing—that is, *constitutional treatment*—the homeopath attempts to find the remedy that will initiate a healing process on the deepest, constitutional level of the entire person.

Frequently, the path to the ultimate remedy requires consecutive prescriptions of other remedies. Each one peels off another layer of problems. It addresses problems that are the most current and disturbing to the mind-body continuum of the patient and therefore the most apparent to the homeopath. Afterward, another layer of problems emerges that requires a different remedy. Each remedy the homeopath selects should be precise and aimed at opening a passageway to the next level of illness and healing.

Even the most experienced homeopaths can face significant difficulties navigating the obstacles of the healing process. As a parent, you shouldn't attempt this type of treatment on your own. Just to give you a brief example, a few years ago, I saw a sixteen-year-old girl named Becky. She told me that she'd run away from home and gone to another state, where she was supposed to meet with representatives of the Mafia, because the CIA, FBI, and a few other important U.S. government agencies wanted her to penetrate it and provide them with information. The mission was so important that Becky lost sleep. But although she was hardly sleeping at all, she still had a lot of energy.

As you can tell, Becky was delusional. The episode had been triggered by the news that her grandmother was becoming progressively ill. Becky loved her grandmother very much. Grandma lived in the city where Becky went to "penetrate the Mafia." When they found her missing, Becky's family had called the police, who were able to catch up with Becky quickly. She was hospitalized in the local psychiatric ward, stabilized on three medications, and then allowed to come home. That's when I met her.

Becky didn't want to take medication for several reasons. First, she was just being a teenager. And she felt good in her delusional state. Second, while on the drugs, her periods were irregular, which was upsetting. Third, Becky read that the medications would cause significant weight gain. That did it. She told her parents that she would have to stop taking them. The parents heard of me and brought Becky to my office.

One of the amazing symptoms that I noticed during the interview was that Becky suffered from psoriasis, a chronic skin disease that's characterized by a particular type of itchy rash. Large areas of her body were covered with the rash. But Becky told me that ever since she'd been "hired by the CIA," the itching had stopped. To me, her situation was obvious. The focus of Becky's problems was much deeper than her skin. It was in the core of her being—at the emotional and mental level. Becky had bipolar disorder.

After a few months of constitutional homeopathic treatment, Becky was able to discontinue taking two out of three of her conventional medications. She remained well. Even though she was a teenager and going to college, Becky did her best over the next several years to follow my directions concerning her lifestyle. Since then, she graduated college and got married. Now we're working together on getting her off her last allopathic medication. She hasn't had any symptoms of mania or depression in all of these years, even under the stress of planning a wedding!

As Becky was getting better, her psoriasis began to itch again. There were also other, new symptoms that led me to prescribe a different remedy. The psoriasis improved by about 80 percent. We hope that after discontinuation of the last conventional drug, Becky's body will be able to get rid of psoriasis completely.

In a way, the difference between the homeopathic treatment of acute and chronic illness is similar to learning a new language. Most of us can navigate ordinary situations during a brief vacation in a foreign country after learning a limited number of words and phrases in a strange language. We don't really need a deep understanding of grammar. We can get by after learning a few basic things about the culture and customs. If we don't understand an answer, we only have to turn to a tour guide for help. Homeopathy for most acute conditions isn't hard to handle, as you'll soon learn in Part Two. If you can't figure it out or you make a mistake, you can always zip over to the ER or phone a doctor.

Constitutional treatment is more like living in a country on a long-term basis. It's a totally different ball game. For that, we need to know the language and culture well. We need to be prepared to react appropriately to every possible situation that we might face. If we didn't have those abilities, we'd have to turn to a knowledgeable guide or partner. In constitutional treatment, homeopaths are the guides and the partners.

Follow-Up Is Very Important

Identifying an appropriate remedy during the first evaluation defines the success of the initial phase of constitutional treatment. But the follow-up appointment with a homeopath is equally important in constitutional care, as new layers of symptoms may emerge once the first remedy has taken effect. The goal is to keep peeling away layers of pathology and restoring the child to the best level of health we can. Children can go from Level Three to Level Two, and from Level Two to Level One, if constitutional treatment works.

Here are a few common scenarios that illustrate why follow-up matters.

Scenario One

The first prescription worked beautifully. All the main complaints went away. The parents therefore decide not to waste their time and money, and they skip the scheduled follow-up appointment.

I know this outcome may sound too good to be true, but it does happen. Children with uncomplicated problems and a high level of health can shake off an illness, such as asthma, relatively quickly provided that the homeopath is able to find the simillimum.

Cases like this keep homeopaths enthusiastic about what we do.

But the road to success can be pretty rocky. Not infrequently, I'll see a child that I saw two or three years earlier, and now the child has another, albeit less severe, problem. It turns out that the child, who originally saw me for, let's say, ADHD, has developed sinusitis after all the symptoms of ADHD have gone away. Even more interesting, the child used to have sinus problems before the ADHD came along. It may be time for a new remedy.

After a main complaint has disappeared, some parents go back to using antibiotics. Then the secondary issue comes back. Or a new problem appears, or the same, severe problem I first treated reappears. Homeopathy to the rescue! But it may be less effective the second time around.

Please come for the follow-up. Don't belittle any health problems your child has. It is better to play it safe and let a specialist see what's going on, and then keep in touch.

Scenario Two

The prescription worked and the main complaint went away. Other severe problems also went away. But there's still a rash of some kind that the child wants to eliminate *now*. The parents decide to treat this "minor" problem allopathically, because that will offer faster relief from the symptoms.

In the case of Becky, for instance, her parents might have decided that because her bipolar disorder was under control, her psoriasis could be treated allopathically. This would have been a major mistake. Fortunately, they didn't do that. Based on what you learned in Chapters One and Two about the four levels of health and about Hering's Law in Chapter One, I'm sure you know that suppressive allopathic treatment of psoriasis may lead to a significant worsening of a child's mental illness, because this approach drives pathology to a deeper level.

My advice is to use homeopathic treatments exclusively, if you can, except in the face of severe physical trauma. Lacerations need to be sewed up and fractures need to be set. In that case homeopathy can be used adjunctively to speed healing. Many times, children, especially teenagers, will nag their parents about pimples on their faces or warts on their feet. If you get nagged, you'll have to be patient. The pimples will fade and the wart will fall off when the time is right. Suppressive treatment of any kind, even for colds or flu, may hold back the curative process and lead to a reversal of the main complaint.

Follow up with your homeopath to determine if there's anything else that can be done for whatever it is that's disturbing your child. The rash may be an aggravation, a sign that healing is under way. Or it may be time for a new remedy.

Scenario Three

Nothing happened after the first prescription—or so the parents think—and therefore they cancel the follow-up appointment, perhaps even without speaking with the homeopath. They are disappointed and assume treatment has failed.

If you base your expectations on someone else's miraculous success story, this action would seem to be appropriate. True, it's amazing that a tiny pill can often quickly turn the life of a very ill child suffering from asthma 180 degrees. In a large number of cases, however, healing takes significantly longer than just a few weeks. Getting to the core issue, which in homeopathy means finding the core remedy, isn't always an easy or straightforward process. There's always a chance that the first remedy your child was given wasn't exactly what was needed at the time. Or there is the possibility that a core issue has indeed improved; but because it's not the one you came for, you haven't noticed that Hering's Law may be working. This doesn't mean that homeopathy has failed. An experienced homeopath will be able to see where to go next.

Finding the right remedy isn't a trial-and-error process. Homeopaths have methods that allow us to eliminate 90 percent or more of the options. Then there's usually a pool of a few possible remedies that are highly likely to be indicated. One of these is the magic key that will open the treasure box and provide the jewel of a cure. The only obstacle is navigating the labyrinth to get to the box. This may be a complicated venture.

Please communicate with the homeopath and go back for your follow-up. Most probably, you won't be disappointed. The lack of an instant resolution of the main issue isn't a sign of incompetence. In chronic illness, there may be many layers to address.

I always marvel at how different the attitude toward conventional care providers is. Parents bring their child with ADHD to an allopathic psychiatrist. He prescribes Ritalin. Let's say there's no effect or there are serious side effects. Rarely would you see anyone simply not coming back and choosing to go to a different doctor. Instead parents go back, get a second prescription, and accept that the side effects are transitory or that they should just give the drug more time to work. And they do. This is normal behavior. I hope you'll be able to think about seeing a homeopath in this rational way, too.

Should You Get a Second Opinion?

There's a famous joke that if you ask two doctors to answer the same clinical question, they will have three different opinions. It's funny because the punch line has a ring of truth to it. If you went to two physicians asking for an antibiotic for your child's sore throat, they might offer you prescriptions for different medications. Needless to say, the situation in homeopathy is even more complex, because there is, in fact, only one correct remedy.

It's good practice for any physician, and certainly for any homeopath, to consult with another health care provider who's seen the same patient. There are situations when a person shows a different doctor a different side, which can make all the difference in the world.

But it is wrong to presume that going to many different homeopaths will increase the chances for better prescribing. The child's presentation of symptoms may change.

If soon after seeing a homeopath, parents bring their child to another homeopath for a second opinion, the second homeopath may prescribe a different remedy. Then a vicious cycle of multiple homeopathic prescriptions can begin. Polypharmacy is never a good idea. Also, parents may get confused and perhaps will therefore seek yet another opinion, only further compounding the problem.

I've even seen cases when a child is brought to different providers in different countries. Of course, the child's presentation can easily change under these conditions, and communication between foreign homeopaths is often difficult. The person who suffers the most from this kind of multiple prescribing is the sick child.

My advice to you is to stick with the same care provider. Homeopaths usually tell you the level of their confidence in the remedy they've chosen for a particular child, and they are happy to discuss the need for a second opinion. If you want to go this route, do it openly, keeping all channels of communication open.

Certain rules apply to all medical professionals. One is that medicine—any form of medicine—is always a combination of art and science.

The majority of homeopaths are hardworking and highly dedicated people. But there may be a rare case when a homeopath seems to be incompetent or strikes a wrong chord with you on a personal level. In this type of situation, for the good of your child, you have to find a new homeopathic care provider in whom you have more confidence.

Should I Ask About a Homeopath's Success Rate?

All homeopaths have been asked about their success rate in treating a particular illness. It's a fair question. But does it have a fair answer? It depends on several factors.

The most important factor in homeopathy is finding the correct remedy. With the exception of severe genetic illnesses and terminal stages of chronic illnesses, every other problem improves or goes away when the simillimum is administered.

What you really should ask are the following:

- *How familiar are you with treating patients with this particular illness?* Even though homeopaths treat individuals, rather than illnesses, having experience with a particular illness does matter. A homeopath must be able to distinguish symptoms common to everyone who has that illness from symptoms unique to your child.

- *How experienced are you in general?* In some cases, such as autism, a crucial element in selecting the right remedy is the ability of the homeopath to pick up on subtle variations of symptoms. This ability only comes with experience.

Both considerations are similar to how you would assess an allopathic physician.

To go back to the issue of success, another important factor is the level of health of a particular patient. Depending on this factor, we may expect either a complete or a partial alleviation of symptoms. Be hopeful, be open-minded, and be realistic.

Using Homeopathy for Acute Ailments When a Child Is Getting Constitutional Care

Most classical homeopaths prefer not to interfere with the course of constitutional treatment by offering children intermediate remedies for mild acute ailments, such as the sniffles or a low-grade fever, especially if there's no change in energy. Your own love and tender care, along with some chicken soup and hot tea, are truly the best medicine in these situations. Of course, in an emergency, you need to intervene.

In the case of a severe cold or flu, contact your homeopath and give the best remedy you can. Then, if the remedy you've chosen doesn't work within a half hour, or the homeopath is not available, promptly seek conventional care.

When your child is receiving constitutional care, you need to reach a very clear understanding with your homeopath on what to do in the case of an acute illness. The majority of parents and homeopaths feel uncomfortable leaving a sick child without any assistance for an extended period of time, and rightfully so.

When Should You Call the Homeopath?

The most logical answer to this question is to call the homeopath whenever your child has an ailment. Unfortunately, reality dictates that there are times when we must deviate from this rule. First of all, you may not be able to reach a homeopath around-the-clock. Ideally, one day soon we'll have homeopathic hospitals in the United States again. But there are none at present. With the possible exception of married couples, the overwhelming majority of homeopaths practice solo, and not all are able to be on call 24/7.

I've faced this issue in my practice for many years. Parents of young children are given my cell phone number, but I shut it down at the end of the day. If a child falls ill during the day, we're in good shape. If not, parents are instructed to use some basic herbs for colds and leave a message so I can call them in the morning.

Sometimes There's No Other Choice

Children are put at great risk when their parents insist on using alternative approaches exclusively and adamantly refuse appropriate conventional treatment. A glaring example would be the rejection of orthopedic help for a child with a fractured arm or leg. Fortunately, I've never seen this extreme a refusal in my own practice.

Now, I can verify that homeopathic treatment significantly reduces the pain and swelling accompanying a bone fracture. Children with broken bones who get homeopathy on the way to the ER often don't look ill at all when they arrive there. They have no pain or swelling. Nevertheless they do have broken bones and definitely require conventional treatment! Broken bones must be set, and the nerves and tissues in the limb must be examined.

In my experience, placing blind faith in a medical miracle usually means that there's underlying fear of a possible diagnosis or of a specific treatment—or both.

I'll never forget the following case: after I had made a presentation during grand rounds at one of the major New York hospitals, a sixteen-year-old high school student named Amy approached me. She'd come to the presentation with her father. They were aware of the success of homeopathy in treating various life-threatening diseases.

Amy had been diagnosed with Hodgkin's lymphoma, a serious cancer that can affect the lymph nodes, spleen, liver, and bone marrow. She was first diagnosed at age fourteen, treated at a prestigious medical institution, but then refused to complete the full course of conventional treatment because she lost her hair. She told me she stopped the chemotherapy, her hair grew back, and she stayed in remission (symptom-free) for about two years. Then her symptoms came back. Although she'd had excellent results from chemotherapy and had a very good prognosis, Amy was refusing the treatment because she didn't want to lose her hair again, even temporarily. Instead she wanted me to treat her homeopathically.

Certainly, there are some reports of great success with homeopathic treatment of various forms of lymphomas. But conventional oncology has an over 85 percent success rate in treating this particular illness. By comparison, the success rate reported by A. U. Ramakrishnan, M.B.B.S., M.F.Hom., Ph.D., the most prominent specialist in homeopathic oncology, is between 50 and 77 percent.

There are no homeopathic oncologists in America. Therefore, the most promising treatment for Amy was appropriate conventional treatment.

After listening to my arguments, Amy and her father, who was totally controlled by this young lady, continued to insist on seeing me. I spent our next two or three consultations trying to convince them to go back to the specialized oncological hospital. To my relief, they finally did.

There are numerous less dramatic, but equally dangerous, examples. A frequently encountered situation is when well-intended parents are completely against conventional medical treatments and antibiotics. Let's say the child of this type of parents develops a sore throat. They don't bring the child to a physician to have him tested for strep throat. Instead they start using homeopathy on their own. If the first remedy they try doesn't work, they try another one, and then another one. No results.

Or let's say the child gets slightly better. He still has residual symptoms, but now without fever. This is a dangerous situation! Untreated sore throat is a condition with a multitude of possible complications.

Of course, an experienced homeopath is able to treat strep throat effectively. An experienced clinician can perform a physical exam and any tests that are necessary to rule out a potentially serious situation. These are steps that parents can't undertake on their own.

For a parent, the best way to cope with strep throat, or any other similar situation, is to head to your physician's office. Maybe you're smart enough and lucky enough to have enlisted the care of a pediatrician or family physician who practices homeopathy. Parents frequently call me in similar situations. My advice is always the same: give your child the best homeopathic remedy you can and seek help right away.

Blind faith will lead you nowhere, even if it is in the power of homeopathy. Yes, it would be preferable to treat your child with homeopathy first, but if you cannot figure out what to do, preventing your child from getting care is a mistake. It's OK. We live in a civilized country where help is widely available. Feel free to admit, "This problem is over my head. Why don't I call my homeopath or physician?"

In the next chapter, we'll take a look at the myths, controversies, and confusion surrounding homeopathy.

Chapter Four

Myths, Controversy, and Confusion

Over the years, much confusion has arisen about the nature of homeopathy. Skeptics continue to attack its theoretical underpinnings. All sorts of unconventional therapies have been lumped together under a single banner, even though many have little to do with the basic principles that define the classical homeopathic approach. Here we'll tackle the skeptics' claims head on and sort through the various healing methods that appear more or less homeopathic.

Let's begin with six familiar misconceptions.

Six Myths About Homeopathy

An enormous amount of commentary about homeopathy is floating around in books by popular authors and on the Internet. Some comes from homeopathic sources. Some comes from those who oppose homeopathy. What makes this flood of information so difficult for a layperson to handle is that the information is often contradictory and it is confusing. If you've been doing research, chances are good that you've encountered the same handful of misconceptions patients usually ask homeopaths to explain.

Myth Number One: Homeopathy Is a Placebo

There's a legend that homeopathy is a *placebo* because it has no side effects and because remedies are delivered to patients on nonactive sugar pellets.[1] But homeopaths know that correctly prescribed remedies for chronic conditions frequently cause an initial, sometimes significant, worsening of the condition—an aggravation. Hahnemann and every homeopath since him have observed this effect. If even the most highly diluted homeopathic remedies are taken too frequently, they result in provings. Healthy, sensitive individuals develop symptoms commensurate with the remedy's picture. (Remember, as discussed in earlier chapters, the remedy that matches a particular set of symptoms constitutes the *picture*.)

If homeopathic remedies were placebos, aggravation symptoms specific to the particular remedy given simply wouldn't occur. This effect shows that remedies are active substances, even though they're highly diluted. But don't confuse an aggravation with a side effect. It's a healing response that quickly passes. It shows that the right remedy was taken. If the wrong remedy is consumed, no effects result.

As for the sugar pellets, remedies don't only come in this form. They can be delivered in the form of tinctures, ointments, tablets, gels, and lotions, too. Please don't confuse the means of delivery with the remedy itself.

By the way, studies show that the placebo effect occurs with every treatment modality. Did you know that even surgery has a high rate of placebo effect? Don't take my word for it. A 1994 article by A. G. Johnson, published in one of the world's most prestigious medical journals, the *Lancet*, illustrates how.[2]

Research has also shown that the positive results of placebos tend to be short-lived. By contrast, homeopathic treatment leaves patients symptom-free for years.

Homeopathy is not a "fake." There's plenty of scientific evidence that it works. Hahnemann's scientific curiosity led him to reject the conventional harmful practices of his own day, much as this book is encouraging you to reject the harmful conventional practices of our day, such as the overuse of antibiotics and steroids. Hahnemann conducted numerous experiments and a thorough search of the professional literature, and these resulted in the discovery of the basic principles of homeopathy. He integrated every progressive discovery of the era, including the discovery of microbes, into his theory. Other scientists largely ignored microbes until Louis Pasteur did his work a few years later.

The nature of homeopathic dilutions remains controversial for conservative allopathic scientists and physicians. Nobody, including homeopaths, likes the fact that to date we can't really understand how and why high dilutions work in the human body. We just can't explain this phenomenon yet. Some remarkable pieces of research suggest that the serial process of dilution and succussion results in the formation of crystalline structures in water that possibly could be the carriers of biological information. But these studies are preliminary. They provide no definitive answer to the mechanism by which ultramolecular homeopathic dilutions produce their healing effect.

In reality, lots of effective medications and therapies don't have well-established mechanisms of action. Clinical results therefore constitute the best jury. And there the verdict is clear: well-designed clinical studies prove homeopathy different from placebo.

At the time of this writing, two meta-analyses of the clinical effects of homeopathy have been published: the first in the *British Medical Journal* (1991), and the second in the *Lancet* (1997).[3] Meta-analysis is research in which data from multiple independent studies on the same subject are pulled together and evaluated collectively. I'm going to get a little bit more technical here to satisfy our most inquisitive readers.

The *British Medical Journal* review assessed 107 controlled trials in 96 published reports. Overall, of the 105 trials with interpretable results, 81 trials indicated positive results versus 24 trials in which no positive effects of homeopathy were found. In studies judged to have better research designs, 15 trials showed positive results, whereas in 7 trials no positive results could be detected. This is significant evidence in favor of homeopathy.

The review in the *Lancet* assessed 186 double-blind or randomized trials (or trials that were both double-blind and randomized). Eighty-nine of these publications had adequate data for meta-analysis. The combined odds ratio was 2.45 in favor of homeopathy. The odds ratio for the 26 good-quality studies was 1.66, and when it was corrected for estimated publication bias (meaning corrected for researchers intent on showing positive results), the ratio remained about the same (1.78). These results are also very significantly in favor of homeopathy's clinical effectiveness.

In other words, homeopathy helps people feel better, which is where it counts.

Nineteenth-century British Prime Minister Benjamin Disraeli once said, "There are three kinds of lies: lies, damned lies and statistics." He had a point. Unfortunately, if someone has his mind set on disproving a scientific claim, or for that matter proving a claim, it is easy to manipulate data in support of that goal. Intentionally, or perhaps unintentionally, researchers have often stacked the deck against homeopathy in the way they design their research protocols. The authors of these studies almost religiously follow this notorious principle: if you ask a silly question, you'll get a silly answer.

Almost each time a study on homeopathy has been designed and carried out by experienced homeopaths, its results have been promising. I know that this statement doesn't come as a surprise. Naturally, one would expect reliable studies on gynecology to be designed by gynecologists, and reliable studies on psychiatry to be designed by psychiatrists, and so on. Please bear these observations in mind each time you do your own literature search and read scientific papers about homeopathy.

A prominent researcher, Daniel Eskinazi, D.D.S., Ph.D., published an interesting paper, entitled "Homeopathy Re-revisited," in the prestigious medical journal *Archives of Internal Medicine* (1999).[4] In it, he demonstrated that if the tenets of homeopathy are restated in modern biomedical parlance, they not only make a lot of sense, they're also fully supported by data from conventional medical textbooks and research.

Myth Number Two: You Have to Believe in Homeopathy for It to Work

This statement presumes that homeopathy is a placebo, and any positive results it produces should be attributed to the power of suggestion. Not so! Every homeopath has handled many cases of skeptical patients coming in prejudiced against homeopathy. They come under the pressure of a spouse or a parent. Homeopathy still works. Believing in it isn't really necessary. It's hard to imagine that merely our best intentions would have been so consistently helpful in curing serious diseases for over two hundred years.

Myth Number Three: Homeopathy Is a Cult That's Frozen in the Nineteenth Century

From functioning as an advanced, scientifically sound branch of medicine during the nineteenth century and early twentieth century, homeopathy was marginalized in America to something similar to a cult during the second half of the twentieth century. This wasn't the case elsewhere in the world—for instance in England, France, Germany, India, South America, and Russia. Due to the rivalry in the United States between those who practice conventional medicine and those who practice homeopathy, the resources of modern science weren't as readily available to homeopaths as to allopaths. There weren't any homeopathic institutions. Medical schools, industry, and the government allocated their resources to a different set of interests.

The problem was compounded by the fact that homeopathic remedies have been in the public domain for so long. Pharmaceutical companies fund a great deal of medical research in this country and elsewhere. But most don't consider the research and development of nonproprietary medications, such as homeopathic remedies, a good financial investment, as remedies cannot be patented and exclusively sold.

One day soon, I hope we will see the re-emergence of full-time homeopathic schools and homeopathic research laboratories. In the meantime, we are blessed with the support of the Samueli Institute for Information Biology, headed by prominent scientist Wayne B. Jonas, M.D. This organization sponsors basic clinical and scientific research on homeopathy and energy medicine. Jonas is a former director of the Office of Alternative Medicine for the National Institutes of Health (NIH) and former director of the Medical Research Fellowship at the Walter Reed Army Institute of Research.

All around the world, scientists like Jonas are conducting research on homeopathy. Two other prominent American researchers are Iris Bell, M.D., Ph.D., and Jennifer Jacobs, M.D. Despite the lack of funds for biomedical research, homeopathic theory and practice have been developing by leaps and bounds. In the last two decades, homeopaths have developed and sharpened new tools for the analysis of patients. For example, homeopaths all use sophisticated homeopathic software now that allows us to cross-reference important symptoms and conduct effective literature searches in minutes. Certainly, this type of analysis requires extensive training in classical homeopathy. A computer cannot find appropriate remedies by itself. But it is a great time-saver.

The homeopathic community has been using new, in-depth approaches to case analysis. Practicing homeopaths spend many hours studying cases and literature. We host numerous national and international professional seminars and conferences. The AIH has an annual meeting. The National Center for Homeopathy (NCH) has an annual meeting. The Liga Medicorum Homeopathica Internationalis (LMHI), an international organization of homeopathic physicians, also conducts meetings annually. There are also many periodic homeopathic publications. Homeopathy is very much alive and advancing.

Although homeopathy went through a dark age of being denied a right to exist, those times are now over. Practitioners of homeopathy, as well as other CAM modalities, are allowed to treat patients and conduct research. Some conventional physicians still assert that homeopaths shouldn't be allowed to conduct research because homeopathy is a "fake." But the National Institutes of Health (NIH) are curious about alternative medicine. Research will do only one thing: help develop reliable homeopathic practice.

Myth Number Four: Homeopathy Is Harmless No Matter What You Do

It's dangerous to believe that homeopathy can be used as frequently as you wish and in any dose. The truth is that homeopathy *only* remains harmless so long as you don't abuse it. But if you follow the advice in this book and only give your child a single dose of one homeopathic remedy at a time, then, yes, homeopathy is safe.

Myth Number Five: Mint Antidotes the Effects of Homeopathy

Old popular books on homeopathy contain the suggestion that mint counteracts—or neutralizes—the effects of remedies. It isn't accurate. What would be accurate is that taking a homeopathic remedy immediately after you've brushed your teeth with mint-containing toothpaste isn't a good idea. The pleasant cool feeling that mint and peppermint produce in the mouth is the result of the constriction of capillaries (small blood vessels). Homeopathy is administered under the tongue to ensure that the remedy gets into the bloodstream as soon as possible. Constricting the blood vessels right before taking the remedy isn't a good idea as it interferes with absorption.

Many homeopathic patients buy special homeopathic toothpaste. These actually contain several homeopathic remedies and might interfere with the progress of treatment. In case you still want to play it safe, there are many kinds of toothpaste without mint. But it's not important. You are welcome to eat mint candies, mint ice cream, and so on.

For some reason, various food items do antidote—or counteract—certain remedies. Your homeopath will know what these are. Certain individuals are more sensitive than others, so it is easier to counteract remedies in such individuals.

In general, remedies are neutralized by allopathic medications; camphor (found in rubs like Tiger Balm and Vicks VapoRub); strong electromagnetic fields (EMFs), such as those emanating from microwave ovens and plug-in alarm clocks; coffee; dental work; and some aromatherapy oils.

Myth Number Six: Homeopathic Remedies Act like Vaccines

Superficially, this statement seems accurate. After all, in both cases it seems as if a person is being given small quantities of a disease in order to avoid the disease. In reality, vaccination and homeopathy are based on similar, but not identical, theories. Homeopathy follows the principle of similars, whereas the same vaccines are given to everyone.

Vaccination stimulates the immune system directly. This process results in the production of antibodies specific to a particular illness. Homeopathy works on a subtler, dynamic level and most probably activates all the body's major integrative systems. Vaccines are tested on animals and are known to cause numerous adverse effects. Homeopathy is tested on humans (provings) and does not have side effects.

This myth leads us to the heart of a debate that's taken place for many years.

Is There Such a Thing as Homeopathic Disease Prevention?

Benjamin Franklin wrote, "An ounce of prevention is worth a pound of cure." All parents understand the wisdom of that expression. Measures designed to prevent disease are called *prophylaxis* and date back to the most ancient of times. People have always wanted protection from the adversities of life, and they've always prayed for the health of their children. As soon as early humans recognized a divine influence, they started creating amulets, or tokens of divine protection. Some carried minerals, gems, and dried animal parts; some carried prayers engraved in stone or on precious metals; others enclosed prayers written on scrolls in leather pouches and other containers. These kinds of prophylaxis continue. Nowadays people frequently wear religious symbols around their necks, or they tie red strings around their wrists and other parts of the body.

The majority of questions about prophylaxis are actually directed toward the prevention of infections. An infection, or an infectious disease, is often defined as a pathological state resulting from the invasion of the body by pathogenic microorganisms (bacteria or viruses). Yet let us rephrase this statement: infection is a result of the *interaction* of the microorganism (bacteria or virus) and the macroorganism (human being). The important point is that a bug is not the same thing as an illness, although it is an important component in disease.

A number of publications have indicated that regular allopathic vaccines and aggressive schedules of their administration could be harmful to children. For that reason, increasingly, parents are seeking so-called homeopathic vaccinations and prophylaxis. Is there any validity to these practices? Is there such a thing as *homeopathic prophylaxis?* Is there such a thing as *homeopathic vaccination?* There is no blanket answer. The truth can be found somewhere in the middle ground.

The situation is clear. To protect our children from infectious disease, we can kill the bugs, we can make our children stronger, or we can do both.

Killing the Bugs

We can destroy bacteria outside the body. This is done by using personal hygiene and sterilization techniques. We can also try to kill or at least weaken microbes that have invaded the body already. That's done with antibiotics or antiviral medications. At the beginning of the twentieth century, when modern biomedical science was established, this approach was popular. It dramatically improved the outcome of surgery. It allowed us to combat infections, such as pneumonia and tuberculosis.

This approach worked well until we noticed that on the one hand bacteria were developing resistance to numerous antibiotics, and on the other hand humans were developing allergic reactions and chronic infections. In addition, it turned out that in the process of killing the real enemy with our powerful antibiotics, we wound up causing enormous collateral damage. We were killing friendly bacteria in the gut that we really need. Antibiotics also weaken our immune system; after all, it is made from cells similar to bacteria. It causes confusion in the parts of the immune system responsible for recognizing the difference between what is "us" (our normal tissues and cells) and what is "foreign" (bacteria, viruses, and sick deformed cells from within the body).

Making Children Stronger

Another preventive approach is to strengthen our children's natural defenses, so they can fight infections more effectively and avoid becoming chronically ill or dying. Parents can participate by using homeopathy for first aid and treatment of mild acute conditions. Homeopaths can offer constitutional treatment to children whose bodies are weaker and more sensitive to the environment. These steps strengthen all of the body's integrative systems, which is the aim of this handbook.

Children also need the following:

- A stable, positive environment
- Physical exercise
- Appropriate rest
- Adequate sleep

- Good nutrition
- Vitamin and mineral supplements (if necessary)
- Love

For homeopathy to help individual children become more resilient to disease, finding a remedy depends on the individual characteristics of a particular child.

In the case of homeopathic prophylaxis, everything depends on identifying a particular disease in a particular population. This is something only a homeopath that sees large numbers of patients can do. It's a public health matter.

In 1801, Hahnemann attended a family with four children during a severe epidemic of scarlet fever. Three of the children contracted the illness. But the fourth and weakest child didn't! Hahnemann remembered that he'd just treated the boy for other problems with *Belladonna*. It was the only difference between him and his siblings. Soon after, Hahnemann attended a family with eight children. Three children had scarlet fever already. He gave *Belladonna* to the other five and they didn't get sick. Hahnemann began giving *Belladonna* to other children with scarlet fever. All were cured. Those who were treated prophylactically didn't get sick. Thus homeopathic prophylaxis was discovered.

Now, despite this success, in later years *Belladonna* wasn't found effective for scarlet fever. A group of homeopathic physicians challenged Hahnemann on this issue. By that time, he'd clearly developed the concept of a *genus epidemicus*: the one remedy that corresponds to the picture of an epidemic illness in a particular population (people in a particular area at a particular time). Once you know the genus epidemicus, you can administer it to individuals within the population to prevent them from developing that illness. It's presumed that this remedy will be used for the duration of the threat.

For example, if there were flu in New York City in November, I might start seeing numerous children requiring *Gelsemium*. My colleagues in New York and New Jersey might also begin to see a number of cases requiring *Gelsemium*. So we'd know that our genus epidemicus was probably *Gelsemium*. In this case, most people in the area could stay well by taking *Gelsemium* 12C every day for the duration of the epidemic.

Come December, we might start seeing a lot of cases that responded to another remedy, let's say *Arsenicum album*. As we begin to see more and more patients cured with *Arsenicum album*, we would realize that the genus epidemicus has changed. *Gelsemium* would no longer be the right remedy to take for prophylaxis.

That's how homeopathic prophylaxis works. It's like finding a group simillimum.

During the terrible flu epidemic of 1918, homeopaths identified three major genus epidemicus remedies. The death rate among people who received one of these remedies prophylactically or who were treated with them was 1.7 percent. Several remedies had to be used because the illness migrated to different geographical regions of the country and infected different populations that were sensitive to different components of the illness.

As you can see, the best preventive homeopathic remedy can be selected only *after* an epidemic begins and homeopaths are able to prescribe the same remedy correctly to a number of people. We truly can't predict ahead of time. Nevertheless the idea that there could be certain remedies for prevention of certain diseases remains popular.

To be clear, homeopathic prophylaxis works only for as long as someone takes the *right* remedy. Usually, homeopaths recommend taking lower potencies (12C or 30C) on a daily basis for the duration of an epidemic. In cases when people don't have any lead time, administration of the remedy will cure most cases of the illness right away. Of course, there are always going to be some exceptions of people who require a different remedy. But the stronger a bug is, the more likely it is that the majority of people in the same region will require the same remedy at the same time.

Homeopathic Vaccination

Now we're ready to talk about the subject of homeopathic vaccination.

Conventional vaccination is a method directed at providing a permanent defense against an infection, one that doesn't require the daily use of medication. Ideally, one or a few applications of a vaccine would provide lifelong protection; though, in reality, boosters are needed for many vaccines.

Vaccinations work in a specific way: by stimulating the immune system to develop antibodies to a particular infection. In the majority of cases, the effectiveness of vaccines can be measured by a test that measures *titers* (or concentration) of antibodies. If titers aren't high enough, it means that the vaccine isn't completely effective. If titers decrease significantly, it means that the person needs a *booster,* another administration of the same vaccine.

It's fair to say that allopathic vaccines hurt a certain population of children. Not everyone is hurt, but some children are. It's also fair to say that vaccines have saved a lot of children. No one on this planet has smallpox anymore. Go ahead and ask your physician when the last time was that she saw a case of diphtheria— probably never. The same is true for polio. Those successes can be attributed to vaccinations.

It certainly would be nice to be able to identify children who potentially could be hurt by vaccinations or even by a particular type of a vaccine. Then we could either treat them constitutionally and vaccinate, or we could not vaccinate them at all. We'd have a choice.

There are at least two questions that we need to answer in relation to this point:

1. Is it possible to prevent side effects of vaccinations with homeopathy?
2. Is it possible to vaccinate children (or adults for that matter) using homeopathic preparations of vaccines?

Preventing Side Effects. Most homeopaths field questions about the prevention of side effects. A lot of parents have heard about using *Thuja, Silicea,* or *Hypericum* for the prophylaxis of side effects from vaccinations. The belief is that if we gave every child, let's say, *Thuja* 200C before vaccination, it would protect all the children from negative side effects, while also allowing their immune systems to develop antibodies. Such a belief is simply false.

The same logic applies to other remedies.

It would be more accurate to presume that children who constitutionally require one of the remedies just listed may be more prone to developing side effects from vaccinations. These children, and only these children, would potentially benefit from these remedies, because, as you know, we are looking for the simillimum, the one right remedy. There is no one-size-fits-all dosing in the classical homeopathic approach.

The best thing parents can do to prevent side effects from conventional vaccinations is to take their children for full homeopathic evaluations and constitutional treatment beforehand. Of course, figuring out what remedy is needed for a baby who can't talk, only consumes mother's milk, and has absolutely no symptoms is very tricky, if not impossible. But if the child is generally sensitive and has various persistent symptoms, such an assessment is possible. Appropriate homeopathic treatment may be helpful in warding off the side effects of vaccinations. It would be nice to be able to conduct such an assessment so early in a child's life, as we could then predict who needs special precautions or treatment.

Another consideration against the use of remedies to prevent side effects from conventional vaccines is that each time there's a vaccination visit to the doctor, the child gets a few shots. Using the same remedy as often as conventional doctors give their shots isn't a good idea at all. It might cause a proving or otherwise derail the child's wellness. And it just contributes to the polypharmacy mixture. Homeopaths are familiar with the so-called confused cases that occur when patients receive multiple doses of homeopathic remedies. Treating these patients is a challenging proposition!

Yet another argument against this type of "prevention" is that there's absolutely no data on whether or not it is efficacious. Anecdotally, some homeopaths recommend it; others don't. Based on what you know about the principles of homeopathy by now, I'm sure you can see that it probably doesn't make too much sense.

It's worth noting that some parents and some medical professionals have questioned the efficacy, safety, and necessity of conventional childhood vaccines since immunization techniques were first conceived. Recently, the term *vaccine-injured children* was used to describe the population of children today who show allergic and other negative reactions to different vaccines. In response to these concerns, homeopathic vaccination methods developed practically alongside conventional vaccination methods.

Beginning with Hahnemann, who introduced them, early homeopaths were interested in using nosodes (homeopathic preparations made from disease tissue) to prevent infectious diseases. Hering later suggested the prophylactic use of *Lyssinum* (homeopathically prepared saliva from rabid dogs) fifty years before Louis Pasteur's famous rabies vaccine. But he never used nosodes himself.

Later homeopaths suggested using specific nosodes for prophylaxis of specific diseases—for example, using *Anthracinum* for anthrax, *Pertussin* for whooping cough, and *Variolinum* for smallpox. If this attractive proposition worked, it would simplify the search for the simillimum. Rather then conducting a full interview and searching for the exact remedy, a homeopath would only need to identify the illness at hand and give out the corresponding nosode.

Can You Use Homeopathic Preparation for Vaccination?
Nosodes were also suggested for use as *homeopathic vaccines*. Today many practitioners and parents have adopted this approach as an alternative to conventional vaccination. According to proponents, homeopathic vaccines induce the immune response and provide protection similar or even superior to conventional vaccines— without side effects. Certainly, homeopathic preparations are less

expensive and don't contain additives, such as mercury, which conventional vaccines do.

I certainly wish things were so simple.

To date, the jury is out on the safety and efficacy of homeopathic vaccines. The idea is closer to allopathic medicine than homeopathy, which is always based on the individualization of treatment. But if something works well and causes no harm, it does not really matter if it is homeopathy, allopathic medicine, prayer, or acupuncture. So we only have to ask this: Is there a sufficient amount of evidence that homeopathic vaccination is effective and harmless? The answer on both points is no.

The main reason we can't answer yes is that the number of well-designed studies on homeopathic vaccination is very small. As a matter of fact, the only well-designed study was conducted on mice by Wayne Jonas, who published his finding in *Alternative Therapies in Health and Medicine* (1999).[5] In this study, 142 male mice were exposed to a deadly disease, tularemia. A standard vaccine protected them in 100 percent of the cases. Nosodes averaged 22 percent. This was better than placebo treatment, under which all of the mice died. Of course, it is only one study, and other studies could produce better (or worse) results.

No one will conduct this type of placebo-controlled studies on humans or even side-by-side studies of homeopathy versus conventional vaccines. But there is some anecdotal evidence from the past. Most of this data was published in homeopathic journals and is difficult to access. For example, a group of authors from Brazil published an interesting paper in the *Journal of American Institute of Homeopathy*.[6] They reported that in 1974 during the outbreak of meningitis in Brazil, 18,640 patients were given the homeopathic nosode *Meningococcinum* as prophylaxis. There were only four cases of meningitis reported in this group. A control group of 6,340 people, who didn't receive any treatment, developed thirty-two cases. The efficacy seems to be obvious.

Conversely, during the 1958 influenza epidemic in Great Britain, 1,100 subjects received homeopathic *Influenzinum* and 500 had no treatment. There was no difference between these two groups in the rate of contracting influenza. In three different studies, conducted in 1932, 1941, and 1946, by various researchers, children developed significant immune response to a homeopathic nosode, *Diphtherinum*. The fact that three independent research groups reproduced the same protocol is significant; however, it is only one study design.

One of the most important reported features of conventional vaccination is that it provides long-term protection after just a few injections, called *booster shots*. A vocal proponent of homeopathic vaccination is Isaac Golden, a homeopath from Australia. He has published books on homeopathic vaccination and has also written an interesting article for *Homeopathy Online*, an Internet publication. According to his recommendations, children have to receive twenty-eight doses of nosodes during the first five years of life.

Golden's schedule is purely arbitrary. There's no particular reason to utilize this, or any other, protocol. He reports that 10 percent of children experience some kind of reaction to the nosodes. Twenty-eight doses of various highly potentized homeopathic remedies may cause significant effects other than the alleged protection from the target illnesses. They actually may create additional long-term health problems that would be difficult to treat with homeopathy. Interestingly, Golden suggests using the nosodes again if an epidemic of one of the target illnesses begins. This means that there's no certainty that children are actually immunized after going through his elaborate protocol.

As you can see, the issue of homeopathic vaccination is complicated. Certainly, the clinical experience of two hundred years demonstrates that genus epidemicus prescribing has always been a forte of homeopathy. It clearly shows impressive results when used according to the principles previously noted. Constitutional treatment also clearly strengthens the defenses of our children and improves their level of health. Furthermore, children born to women who were treated with homeopathy during pregnancy are reported to be healthier. However, no controlled research studies on this subject are available.

Now you have sufficient information to draw your own conclusions.

What Homeopathy Is

Classical homeopathy is a term coined to distinguish homeopathy practiced according to the original principles discovered by Hahnemann from everything else. The majority of American homeopaths practice classical homeopathy. This handbook is based on the classical homeopathic approach, which has three main features:

- The principle of similars
- Minimal dose
- Single remedy

Pluralistic homeopathy is another form of homeopathy, which is popular in France. Pluralists use frequent dosing, and they alternate different remedies throughout the day. Unlike classical homeopathy, this approach is deeply focused on pathology—changes that can be perceived—with a significant emphasis on concrete changes observed during the physical exam. The patient is kept busy taking medication. At times, people are asked to take up to ten different remedies in different concentrations at different times of the day.

Certainly, classical homeopaths disapprove of these prescribing practices, although pluralists are known to get decent results. In classical theory, the effect of multiple remedies and frequent dosing is suppressive. However, I know a few well-trained pluralists who actually use single remedies most of the time despite their background.

Regionally, homeopaths differ in regard to the potencies they use. The majority of North American homeopaths use centesimal dilutions (for example, 30C, 200C). Usually, the higher a dilution one uses, the less frequently one needs to take it. By contrast, homeopaths from Argentina and some other countries use decimal dilutions (for example, 3X, 6X). These preparations are taken a few times a day.

In many cases, modifications of homeopathy lead practitioners to deviate from the basic principles that make homeopathy most effective. Their so-called improvements and advances may actually render these new methods nonhomeopathic and ineffective; however, no comparative studies have been done. Essentially, these variations involve using homeopathic remedies in an allopathic manner. So far, the clinical results of these "innovative" methods haven't been as impressive as for classical homeopathy.

Interestingly, the future of allopathic medicine itself seems to lie in the direction of *differential therapeutics*, a term for utilizing more individualized treatment of patients, for instance, for cancer. It's clear to everyone that different people respond with variations to the same medication. In prescribing conventional drugs, some doctors try to harness side effects to assist their patients' secondary complaints. For instance, if two patients have been diagnosed with the same disease, but one is lethargic and the other has insomnia, and there's a medication for the disease that in addition to its intended action also induces drowsiness, the doctor may give it to the insomniac patient. Why not make use of it?

Homeopathic Combination Remedies

The most prominent items in the homeopathic section of most health food stores are the so-called combination remedies. They are definitely best-sellers. These products seem to offer a simple and straightforward solution: one medication for one diagnosis. We can find combination remedies for almost anything that ails us, conditions ranging from teething, to head colds, to premenstrual syndrome, to hemorrhoids. Combination remedies exist on the border of homeopathy and allopathic medicine, because they are efficacious, like other homeopathic approaches, but they are prescribed for a condition and not for an individual. They're also examples of homeopathic polypharmacy. Most important, at times they provide very efficacious, temporary symptom relief while the body cures itself.

Are these remedies good? Some are useful for self-limiting conditions in strong children—those with Level One or Level Two health. The major homeopathic companies use combinations that have been tested for years and have been shown to be effective, but to reiterate, only for the *temporary* relief of self-limiting conditions. Treating serious or chronic conditions with combination remedies isn't a good idea.

The idea of combination remedies seems to be very simple. Two or more remedies known to relieve a particular symptom, or sometimes an illness, are combined in the same tablet. The expectation is that either the action of the combination will be synergistic (meaning that the remedies will enhance one another) or that at least one of the remedies will be exactly what the patient needs.

Frederick Humphreys, M.D., a homeopath who was expelled from the AIH and the New York State Homeopathic Medical Society for using these remedies, introduced combination remedies into practice in 1885. He created them to reconcile the homeopathic and allopathic approaches, an impossible proposition. He hoped that there would be specific remedies for certain illnesses. But the premise is wrong. In homeopathy, we treat the whole person. We base prescriptions on the indicators that make people different from one another, rather than on the symptoms that make everyone the same. What combination remedies do instead is to offer a quick fix to the public.

Setting that erroneous notion aside, we also know that any type of polypharmacy is considered to be highly undesirable in both homeopathic and allopathic medicine. Do you recall the story about the lobster, stork, and donkey pulling in different directions?

Another common mistake is calling a remedy homeopathic just because it was diluted and potentized. A remedy is actually considered homeopathic only because of the manner in which it is being used. In order to be used homeopathically, the substances don't have to be diluted or shaken. Early homeopaths used drops of pure tinctures. The main feature of homeopathy is the application of medicinal substances according to the principle of similars. Hahnemann clearly said in his main work, *Organon of the Medical Art*, "In no case of cure is it necessary to employ more than a single simple medicinal substance at one time with a patient."[7]

Some combination remedies are effective for temporary relief of symptoms. There are impressive combination remedies that palliate vertigo, inflammation, and teething. If you're going to use combination remedies, please remember that use should be limited and it might be suppressive. Any claim that a company has found an "easy solution" is not accurate at all. Real healing requires an understanding of individual traits.

An important consideration is whether or not combination remedies can damage your child. If your child has Level One or Level Two health, most probably he or she will either benefit from a short course of, let's say, a teething combination, or nothing at all will happen. A combination remedy might harm a child who is weaker and more sensitive.

As a general rule of thumb, don't use combination remedies if your child is under the care of a professional homeopath. These preparations, as well as other medications, might interfere with the progress of constitutional treatment.

Cell Salts (Tissue Salts)

Cell salts have been presented to consumers as a different type of medicine than homeopathy, although in truth they are homeopathic preparations. They are sold in many health food stores, sometimes without a detailed description of what they are made from. Some parents believe that if they give cell salts to their children, they can speed up their kids' growth, cure their sinus problems and other chronic infections, and help them overcome sleep disorders. Bottom line, cell salts are marketed as medicine in their own right, but they are an extension of homeopathy. They are only effective medicine, however, if they're prescribed by a homeopath who's utilizing the principle of similars. Parents should not prescribe cell salts for their own children.

Cell salts are made from some of the chemical elements found inside the cells of the human body. They are also found elsewhere in nature. German physician Wilhelm Schuessler introduced them in 1873. He erroneously thought he had found a new principle of cure. But he denied any connection with homeopathy. His original article, published in German, went unnoticed until a small book by Constantine Hering, entitled *Twelve Tissue Remedies*, was published in May 1873. Then Schuessler witnessed twenty-five editions of his book get printed before his death in 1898. In the later editions, he denied any connection between his method and homeopathy. He insisted that his method was based only on the biochemistry of the human cell.

Schuessler's theory was based on the idea that the structure and vitality of the organs of the human body are dependent upon certain quantities of minerals present in human cells. His theory had no experimental basis. Cell salts are homeopathically prepared, usually in potencies of 3X, 6X, 12X, and 30X. He used most of the salts in 6X and only a few at 12X. His biochemical theory also talks about the content of the cell salts in various homeopathic remedies. What makes cell salts unique is that they are prepared all the way by trituration. As you may recall, trituration is the process Hahnemann devised to convert insoluble materials into a form that could be introduced into the core process of dilution and succussion. In classical homeopathy, triturations are only used for the first three steps of the attenuation process.

Schuessler suggested the use of twelve preparations. Modern homeopathic companies sell fourteen. The two additional ones are combinations. One of them is called *bioplasma*. It contains all twelve cell salts: nine in 3X, and the remaining three in 6X. Another combination is called *biochemic phosphates*. It contains only the five salts that contain phosphates. According to the proponents of this combination, it's supposed to be good for the nervous system. All the remedies in this combination are 3X.

Schuessler subscribed to the individualization of treatment, and actually there is a short cell salt repertory available in various editions of his work, as well as in books on the methodology of cell salt treatment. All twelve cell salt remedies are also used as regular homeopathic preparations in the practice of classical homeopathy. But classical homeopaths do not subscribe to Schuessler's biochemical theory. We simply happen to use preparations made from the same materials because most of them existed *before* Schuessler. For example, *Calcarea salts* and *Silicea* are homeopathic remedies first described by Hahnemann. Although slow acting, cell salts shouldn't be used without control or appropriate advice from trained homeopaths. The prophylactic use of cell salts is of questionable value, both from the therapeutic and safety points of view.

What Homeopathy Isn't

Homeopathy is everything that uses the principle of similars. Everything else is not homeopathy. Methods described in this section aren't necessarily "bad" practices; some are quite efficacious, such as herbal medicines. They just aren't homeopathy. Frequently, medical treatment is mysterious. Although mystery may be appealing to some, my view is that having a clear understanding of what is going on or not going on during any treatment is important for ensuring the safety of children.

Herbal Medicine

A large number of people come to my office with the mistaken belief that homeopathy and herbal medicine are the same. In fact, they are like apples and oranges. Homeopathic remedies are potentized and must be administered one at a time. By contrast, herbs are neither diluted nor succussed, and herbal medicines are often administered several at a time. In addition, homeopathic remedies are made from various natural substances, which include, but are not limited to, herbs. In general, herbs are used, just as conventional pharmaceuticals, for the biochemical properties of their constituents.

Bach Flower Remedies

Many people considered the Bach Flower Remedies to be part of the field of homeopathy. They are not. Dr. Edward Bach (pronounced *batch*) started his career as a bacteriologist and pathologist at the London Homeopathic Hospital. Homeopathy became his main interest, and in 1926 he coauthored a book on homeopathy. He was also interested in plants. In 1930, he left London and went to the countryside to investigate the healing power of flowers. He ultimately developed thirty-eight flower essences. Although frequently referred to as homeopathic, these interesting and effective remedies are not homeopathic in the way they are prepared, nor in the way they are used for treatment.

Bach rejected the cornerstone principle of similars. He believed in natural beauty, and he believed that good replacing evil would lead to "true healing." He also believed that diseases could be eliminated only by spiritual and mental effort. He described thirty-eight states of diseased soul and mind and offered a remedy for each. Bach placed the main emphasis of cure on self-realization and spiritual progress.

About the flower essences, he stated that the action "is to raise our vibrations and to open up our channels for the reception of Spiritual Self."[8] His two main methods of preparation of his remedies were exposure to the sun and boiling. Although he called these methods potentization, they obviously differ significantly from homeopathy.

According to many witnesses, Bach was an amazing healer. Always frail, he died in his sleep at age fifty. Bach remedies remain very popular. There's plenty of anecdotal evidence of their efficacy. But one thing is clear: they aren't homeopathy.

Anthroposophic Medicine

Austrian philosopher-scientist Rudolf Steiner founded a spiritual movement called *anthroposophy*, which incorporates a medical approach. He viewed humans as a system of four interconnected parts. He suggested that the *physical body* is related to minerals. The life force, called the *etheric body* by him, is related to plants. And the *astral body*, represented by the emotions and the soul, is related to animals. According to Steiner, the human system also possesses a fourth important component: the *ego*.

Anthroposophic medical treatment is highly individualized and only sometimes utilizes homeopathically prepared remedies. In addition, medications are prescribed according to principles different from those of classical homeopathy.

Homotoxicology

German physician Hans Heinrich Reckeweg formulated *homotoxicology* in 1952, presenting it as an attempt to create a missing link between homeopathy and allopathic medicine. In homotoxicology, diluted and potentized preparations are administered according to both allopathic indications and theoretical principles set forth by Reckeweg. He suggested that illnesses are caused by direct toxic influences of various substances and *non-material*. By this, he meant influences like electromagnetic fields and psychic energy. He called influences *homotoxins*.

Reckeweg further hypothesized that homotoxins interact with one another or are processed in the liver to neutralize them. He called homotoxins that aren't eliminated through this process *retoxins*. Combined with homotoxins, these can affect the cells and tissues of the human body, triggering a process called *homotoxicosis*.

The goal of Reckeweg's treatment is to eliminate homotoxins and assist the cells and tissues in elimination of retoxins deposited in their membranes. To accomplish these purposes, homotoxicology uses various preparations, including homeopathic remedies, conventional medications that are homeopathically prepared, enzymes, nosodes, and what are called *Suis-organ* preparations (homeopathically prepared organs and tissues of healthy pigs). Medications are administered both orally and through injections. This type of treatment is most probably suppressive in its action.

Homotoxicology is an attempt to use potentized remedies allopathically. But it isn't homeopathy in any shape or form. It has gained popularity with integrative physicians and their patients, and it's been incorporated into the more complex field of biological medicine, which draws upon elements of holistic dentistry, chelation (a therapy that uses IVs purportedly to cleanse your blood and body), Western medicine, Eastern medicine, and homeopathy. At present, there's no evidence of its efficacy or lack thereof. Please remain aware of the risks of combining medications.

Homotoxicologists use injectable homeopathic remedies. Although these are potentized preparations of various substances, they don't represent homeopathy. Are they effective? Possibly. But if they are, they aren't different from allopathic medications. I'm not necessarily saying that they aren't helpful. Injectables are not homeopathy, that's all.

Homeopathic Drainage

French physician Léon Vannier developed *homeopathic drainage* between 1911 and the 1950s. This revisionist method of homeopathy is more popular in Europe than in the United States. It is based on a hypothesis, rather than on direct research data, that presumes that the main issue in the disease process is the accumulation of toxins in the body. It also incorporates polypharmacy, which is highly undesirable. Homeopathic drainage employs many homeopathic remedies simultaneously.

Vannier insisted that the choice of the drainage remedy should be individualized. In his process, the patient receives a *fundamental remedy*, which is selected based on a concept that's analogous, but not identical to, the concept of the simillimum. On top of that, a nosode is always prescribed as a *regulating remedy*. Then there are one or two *drainage remedies* in low potency, as well as *lesional remedies* directed toward regional problems. As a result, a patient may be receiving two remedies in high dilutions (200C), two in medium (30C), and one or two in low dilutions (6C). Remedies are usually administered in monthly cycles in increasing dilutions. They may also be changed according to the changes of symptoms.

Vannier also invented so-called *prenatal homeopathy*, by which he meant something quite different than giving health care to pregnant women. Essentially, he suggested that instead of waiting for a child to be born with systemic conditions, one could administer nosodes to a pregnant mother to protect her child from future illnesses. He insisted that DNA could be modified in this way and hereditary disease prevented. Unfortunately, there are no data to support or detract from this hypothesis.

Electrodiagnostic Machines

Some practitioners use *electrodiagnostic* devices to select homeo-pathic remedies. Proponents claim that the cause of disease is an energy imbalance that can be detected. They say such devices can diagnose diseases, including allergies and food sensitivities, vitamin deficiencies, asthma, cardiac problems, and even cancer and AIDS. Although they employ remedies, they often prescribe more than one, and in various potencies. They also use the devices to test the patient's need for supplements and allopathic medications.

In the early days, there was no computer present in this diagnostic system. The early devices were called *Voll machines*, and the procedure itself was called *electro-acupuncture according to Voll* (EAV) or *electrodermal screening* (EDS). German physician Reinhold Voll developed the first device in 1958 so he could com-bine Chinese acupuncture theory with galvanic skin differentials in his system.

The main part of any EAV system is a galvanometer that mea-sures the electrical resistance of the patient's skin when touched by a probe. The device emits a very low voltage (frequently below one volt) direct electric current. A first wire from the device is con-nected to a brass cylinder that's covered by moist gauze. The patient holds this in one hand. A second wire is connected from the device to a probe, which the operator touches to various acupuncture points on the patient's other hand or a foot. This completes a low-voltage circuit and the device registers the flow of current.

The device is said to indicate the condition of a particular meridian or energy channel and its corresponding organs. This information is relayed to a gauge that provides a numerical readout on a scale of 0 to 100. Readings below 45 suggest organ stagnation and degeneration. Readings from 45 to 55 are considered normal and balanced. Readings above 55 indicate inflammation of the organ associated with the meridian being tested. The circuit includes a honeycomb cache in which glass ampoules holding various preparations can be placed to correct for supposed deficiencies. The operator then observes changes on the dial and knows what remedy is indicated.

The original technique required examination of up to 850 acupuncture points. Then one of the Voll's students, Helmut Schimmel, simplified the diagnostic system, made small modifications to the equipment, and created a new model, known as a *Vegatest*. There are many such devices on the market currently. All of them utilize computers. Nowadays this technique is called *bioelectric functions diagnosis* (BFD), *bioresonance therapy* (BRT), or *bioenergy regulatory technique* (BER).

A complete examination for asthma or allergies may involve testing up to sixty acupuncture points and involves miraculous readings for viral, bacterial, and chemical toxins. Then the computer suggests a list of potentially effective substances for treatment, including single and combination homeopathic remedies, nosodes, allergens, herbs, vitamins, minerals, and other items. These substances are then tested individually to determine which ones would allow the patient's body to return to a state of energetic harmony. Obviously, the ultimate prescription contains numerous components, including various homeopathic preparations.

The equipment is expensive. The evaluation is impressive and projects a flavor of real science and technology, with multicolor schematic readouts on a computer screen. But this method is not homeopathy. Furthermore, its efficacy hasn't been adequately tested in controlled studies, and the ultimate treatment involves polypharmacy.

In Part Two, you'll learn the basics for successfully using homeopathy to treat the acute health problems of your child.

Part Two

Treating Acute Health Problems

Chapter Five

Basic Remedies for Your Home Homeopathic Kit

Homeopathy is extremely effective in the treatment of acute conditions, as it aborts the development of a vicious cycle of serious, long-lasting problems. Rather than turning you into a professional homeopath, the goal of this chapter is to provide you with a quick reference source, a brief introduction to sixty-three useful remedies. A large number of homeopathic self-help books have been published since the 1980s. Usually, these books contain incredibly detailed information on numerous remedies and teach their readers how to prescribe for acute and even chronic conditions. Once this was necessary. Two decades ago, there were few experienced homeopaths in the United States. Today, twenty-five years later, the situation is very different. You don't need to become your children's homeopath anymore, as you can easily consult one. There are many good homeopaths in this country and around the world. They're trained to heal people.

Your Homeopathic Kit

You'll need to have homeopathic remedies at home in order to save time in an emergency or whenever an acute condition arises, as the earlier you use a remedy, the better a result you can expect to see. Numerous remedies are now sold in health food stores and in some of the more enlightened drugstores, but frequently the potency of the remedies on the shelf isn't what you need or the selection of remedies in the store is limited, so it's essential to plan ahead. It's important to have the remedy at hand—in the right potency—when your child is getting sick. I therefore suggest building your own homeopathic kit according to the following recommendations.

For the same reasons, it's also a very good idea to carry a small remedy kit that contains a selection of any special remedies you might need when you travel.

You can either buy single remedies through your local health food store, pharmacy, or online supplier, or you can mail order a prepackaged Dr. Shalts' AIH Remedy Kit for Parents (see Resources section). Retailers can always order remedies in the potencies you request if they don't have them on hand.

Your kit should contain all of the remedies in the following list, including tinctures and ointments. As you've already learned, the picture of each homeopathic remedy has many indications. Furthermore, homeopathic remedies are multidimensional—meaning, they have many applications. Here you'll find concise descriptions of the few characteristics you may need to know to make a quick, effective decision in the case of an emergency.

Remember, in homeopathy each individual may need a different remedy. There can be several possible remedies for the same ailment. This book only provides general guidelines for home-based homeopathy. In future chapters, I'll remind you of the most prominent characteristics of each remedy that must clearly be present before you prescribe it under specific circumstances. You can also easily obtain more information.

The characteristics that are outlined in the following list are accurate, and they'll give you a strong "backbone" for any future research.

1. *Aconitum napellus* (monkshood). One of the main homeopathic remedies, it's used for many acute conditions. The state of the person who needs it can be described in one word: *terror*. The main characteristic of symptoms that respond to *Aconitum* is sudden, violent, disastrous onset with a feeling of extreme panic. Other indications are experiencing sudden high fever while feeling

hot, having severe thirst for cold drinks, feeling scared, and experiencing restlessness. This remedy is beneficial for many people who witness or survive natural disasters and terrorist attacks. A child with a sudden onset of a cold who needs *Aconitum* would be scared and restless.

2. *Aethusa cynapium* (fool's parsley). *Aethusa* is one of the best friends of breast-feeding babies. It is almost a specific remedy for babies who vomit large curds of milk after each feeding. Babies who benefit from *Aethusa* frequently lack thirst. They also frequently have diarrhea and are weak, exhausted, and don't sleep well (things expected from hungry babies).

3. *Allium cepa* (red onion). Just imagine the way you feel when you peel an onion: you cry bland tears and have an irritating discharge that comes out of your nose (compare with *Euphrasia officinalis*, which reverses these two symptoms), and you also sneeze frequently. If you keep peeling the onion longer, you feel a heavy, stupefying sensation in your forehead and your throat feels raw. *Allium* is helpful in treating acute hay fever, colds, laryngitis, and sinusitis.

4. *Anacardium orientalis* (marking nut). This interesting remedy ameliorates many different physical and emotional conditions. Homeopaths use it to treat some forms of nausea that occur during pregnancy and many cases of poison ivy.

5. *Antimonium crudum* (black sulphide of antimony). This is an interesting multipurpose remedy, which is difficult at times to distinguish from *Chamomilla*. Homeopaths often use it for the treatment of chicken pox.

6. *Antimonium tartaricum* (tartar emetic). Children who need this remedy frequently have bronchitis, characterized by a wheezing cough with mucus bubbling and rattling in their chest. The child is pale and looks very sick.

7. *Apis mellifica* (honeybee). This remedy relieves most symptoms caused by insect bites and bee stings. It can also be helpful any time there's significant swelling accompanied by heat and redness. Compare it with *Ledum*.

8. *Arnica montana* (leopard's bane). Many homeopaths say that if people only could learn about one remedy, they'd teach them about *Arnica*. It's a major remedy for any type of blunt trauma or surgery that damages both the soft tissues and bone structures. That's why I carry *Arnica* 10M in my bag and keep it in the glove compartment of my car. An indicator is that someone frequently complains of a sore, bruised feeling. *Arnica* should come to mind whenever there's been a significant accident or a serious fall. This is especially so if your child is convinced of being OK despite severe consequences of trauma. Interestingly, hours later someone who needs *Arnica* reports feeling scared of the accident that happened.

A note of caution is this: for all its benefits, *Arnica* is also the most overused homeopathic remedy. Please don't give it each time your child falls, and don't give your child frequent repeat doses, as these may cause a proving.

9. *Arsenicum album* (oxide of arsenic). This remedy made it into a best-selling book! In 1999, Chris Bohjalian published a novel, *The Law of Similars*, in which Chapter Nine is entitled *Arsenicum album*. How would you feel about giving poison to your beloved child? That's exactly how people who need this remedy feel: extremely anxious and restless, with upset stomachs and diarrhea. They're also thirsty for small sips of cold water. *Arsenicum* is almost a specific for food poisoning. It's also frequently prescribed for the treatment of chronic problems. *Arsenicum* is a *polychrest* (a remedy that has many widespread uses).[1] It can be helpful for more than ten thousand symptoms!

10. *Belladonna* (deadly nightshade). This is a major remedy for the treatment of acute conditions. As in the picture of *Aconitum*, symptoms come on suddenly and forcefully. But in contrast with *Aconitum*, usually the person who needs *Belladonna* is confused and lethargic, with enlarged pupils. Often the head is hot and the face is flushed. The hands and feet are cold.

11. *Bellis perenis* (common daisy). This is a very useful remedy for trauma to the internal organs. It's beneficial for bruises and swelling that last a long time.

12. *Bryonia alba* (white bryony). This is yet another major remedy for acute ailments. In older books, people who need *Bryonia* are described as "grumpy bears," as they're usually irritable and want to be left alone. Even the slightest motion causes severe pain and discomfort. To understand the *Bryonia* state, imagine how someone who just broke a bone might feel: afraid to move and also trying to reserve every tiny bit of energy that's left. Whatever the ailment is—a cold, flu, headache, or anything else—the child who benefits from *Bryonia* feels much worse from movement and is very thirsty for large quantities of cold water.

13. *Calendula officinalis* (marigold). This remedy could easily be named a homeopathic *water of life*, as its preparations (ointment, tincture, or pellets) are so useful for stimulating the healing of cuts and surgical wounds.

14. *Cantharis* (Spanish fly). This remedy has many applications, one being acute urinary tract infections. In this book, we'll talk about its use for minor burns.

15. *Carbo vegetabilis* (vegetable charcoal). An amazing remedy that could be described as the *reviver*. It helps in cases of collapse and severe weakness when people are made significantly better by being fanned or having fresh air from any source blown in their faces.

16. *Carbolicum acidum* (carbolic acid). This interesting remedy will be discussed in Chapter Six as a remedy for bites of poisonous insects and snakes.

17. *Caulophyllum thalictroides* (blue cohosh). This remedy is homeopathy's gift to women who are about to birth their babies. It does miracles in cases of protracted, painful labor. Native Americans call cohosh *birth root*.

18. *Causticum* (potassium hydrate). This was one of the major homeopathic remedies first introduced by Hahnemann. We'll explore using it for the treatment of a dry cough that gets better in rainy weather and from drinking cold liquids in Chapter Six. It's appropriate if a child wants to cough up something in his chest, but it won't come out. The cough vanishes during the day.

19. *Chamomilla* (German chamomile). One of the best friends of parents who have to deal with cranky babies, *Chamomilla* is almost a specific for painful teething. It also works miracles for those who are hypersensitive to pain.

20. *Coccus cacti* (cochineal). This remedy is used for dry, spasmodic coughs that get worse in warm rooms and improve from cold air and cold drinks.

21. *Cocculus indicus* (Indian cockle). *Cocculus* is one of the main remedies for motion sickness.

22. *Coffea cruda* (unroasted coffee). Homeopathically prepared coffee does exactly the opposite of the crude substance. It helps overly excited people to calm down and go to sleep. Although it's very useful for acute situations, make sure that you don't wind up giving it to your child every night for several days in a row. If the problem persists after a few doses of this remedy, consult a homeopath.

23. *Colchicum autumnale* (meadow saffron). Another homeopathic gift for pregnant women, this remedy is frequently used for gout, and it also resolves some cases of morning sickness, especially when even a thought of food can make a mother-to-be feel nauseous.

24. *Colocynthis* (bitter cucumber). This remedy is often useful for colic. Children (and adults) who benefit from *Colocynthis* feel better with *hard pressure* and from *bending double*. Signs that it's appropriate are that a child's pain can be provoked or gets worse from anger, and the child is usually restless with pain. Compare this remedy with *Magnesia phosphorica*. In addition, please note that individuals made better by bending backward (rather than forward) benefit from *Dioscorea villosa* (wild yam), which isn't on this list, as it is so infrequently indicated.

25. *Cuprum metallicum* (copper). It's a very useful remedy for many conditions that involve spasms.

26. *Drosera rotundifolia* (sundew). *Drosera* is famous for its use as a treatment for coughs, especially whooping cough. The most characteristic symptom is a cough so severe that children have paroxysms during which they cannot catch their breath and may become cyanotic. Frequently, children also have nosebleeds or

vomit as a result of this cough, which is made worse by eating. Another characteristic is worsening immediately upon lying down at night.

27. *Dulcamara* (bittersweet). Any ailment that's been brought about by damp, cold weather should make you think about using this remedy.

28. *Eupatorium perfoliatum* (boneset). This remedy is very useful in cases of flu and colds where people are complaining of a pain in their bones, as if the bones were broken. Frequently, people who need it also complain of severe back pain. They have fever preceded by chills and a paradoxically severe thirst for cold drinks.

29. *Euphrasia officinalis* (eyebright). *Euphrasia* is a very useful remedy for bouts of hay fever in which the tears are irritating and nasal discharge is bland. (Remember that *Allium cepa* fits exactly the reverse of these two symptoms.)

30. *Ferrum phosphoricum* (phosphate of iron). This important remedy is useful in the treatment of colds, flu, and earaches. The child who needs it usually has a high fever, but no other local symptoms, and the onset of the fever is often gradual. It's not as dramatic a picture as the picture for *Aconitum*.

31. *Gelsemium sempervirens* (yellow jasmine). For many reasons, this is a significant remedy. You will see a need for it in some cases of cold and flu, and also for acute anxiety and stage fright. Children who need *Gelsemium* for colds and flu feel weak, complain of having a heavy head, and may say that they're having difficulty keeping their eyes open.

32. *Glonoine* (nitroglycerin). Constantine Hering discovered the medicinal use of nitroglycerin. It has many interesting applications. We will utilize it for heat strokes.

33. *Hamamelis virginiana* (witch hazel). This remedy can be helpful to pregnant women suffering from varicose veins. For this purpose, I usually recommend a low potency of 6C.

34. *Hepar sulphuris calcareum* (calcium sulfate). This is one of the most frequently used remedies for croup, ear infections, and numerous other problems. Children who benefit from it often are

absolutely intolerant of cold drafts and cold environments. They may complain of feeling worse when even a part of their body is uncovered or when simply touching a cold bottle from the refrigerator. On the emotional level, these children can be very irritable. Extreme sensitivity on all levels is the key symptom.

35. *Hydrastis canadensis* (golden seal). Well known for its use in treating sinusitis, an important characteristic of this picture is a marked postnasal drip. *Hydrastis* is indicated when nasal discharge is copious and thick. People who need it usually are constipated. Compare it with *Kali bichromicum*, noting that those who need *Kali* frequently have deep nasal voices and complain of diarrhea.

36. *Hypericum perforatum* (St. John's wort). Some homeopaths call this remedy "Arnica for the nerves." It relieves pain from injuries to the parts of the body that are reached by the nerve endings, such as fingertips and toes and the tailbone. It has helped many children whose fingers got caught in doors, even if the digits were crushed.

37. *Ignatia amara* (St. Ignatius' bean). *Ignatia* is a major remedy for grief (for example, from the loss of a pet or a breakup). One of the chief symptoms of this picture is a frequent sigh. Teenagers swear by it, as it helps "repair" their broken hearts. I've also given this remedy prophylactically to people just before a funeral.

38. *Ipecacuanha* (ipecac root). This remedy relieves severe nausea and severe cough or croup associated with vomiting. It is also very helpful for a combination of nausea with bleeding from any part of the body when the blood is bright red and comes out in gushes, as can happen immediately after giving birth.

39. *Kali bichromicum* (potassium bichromate). This is a remedy for acute sinusitis when there is a gluey, thick green or yellow discharge from the nose and someone's voice sounds nasal. The person may complain of heaviness and burning at the root of the nose. There might also be a headache (characteristically in one small spot) and photophobia, or light sensitivity. If there is any problem with the stools, it's usually diarrhea. Compare this remedy with *Hydrastis canadensis*.

40. *Lachesis muta* (bushmaster snake venom). Also discovered by Constantine Hering, this is an amazing remedy that has saved the lives of thousands of stroke victims and is also used for many other indications. In this book, we'll recommend it only for people who travel in places infested with snakes.

41. *Ledum palustre* (marsh tea). An important remedy for animal bites; stings from large insects, such as wasps; and puncture wounds. The site of such a wound is characteristically cold to the touch and swollen, and the person feels much better from cold applications—so much so, in fact, that children who need *Ledum* probably won't want to let go of an ice pack. Children who need this remedy may be chilly; nonetheless they get better from ice-cold applications.

42. *Magnesia phosphorica* (phosphate of magnesia). This remedy relieves spasmodic pains, as in leg cramps, menstrual cramps, and colic, which are made much better from warm applications and bending over double. Unlike in the picture for *Colocynthis*, hard pressure is not as helpful as warm applications.

43. *Mercurius iodatus flavus* (protoiodide of mercury). This and the next remedy are related. *Flavus* is very useful when the symptoms of a sore throat are strongly presented on the right side.

44. *Mercurius iodatus ruber* (biniodide of mercury). *Ruber* is a left-sided relative of the previous remedy. It is almost a specific for an acute left-sided sore throat.

45. *Mercurius solubilis* (or *vivus*) (quicksilver). This remedy is a polychrest that's useful in cases of common colds, tonsillitis, and ear infections. Children who need this remedy are very sensitive to temperature changes (reminiscent of mercury thermometers). They perspire a lot, are weak, and have trembling hands. In addition, they have offensive breath and their tongues have imprints from their teeth. They also drool and their lymph nodes are enlarged.

46. *Nux vomica* (Quaker button). *Nux* is another polychrest and can help your child fight headaches, flu, and digestive problems. It would be a favorite remedy of college students if they knew how helpful it is for hangovers or any kind of overindulgence in food.

47. *Oxalicum acidum* (oxalic acid). This remedy should become a part of the kit for people who expect to be in places infested with snakes and large poisonous insects.

48. *Petroleum* (crude rock oil). This remedy is useful for some cases of car sickness.

49. *Phosphorus* (phosphorus). Also a polychrest, this remedy is helpful for the treatment of vomiting when even a small gulp of water is almost immediately thrown up, as well as for chest colds and some forms of bleeding.

50. *Phytolacca decandra* (poke root). Great American homeopath James Tyler Kent called this remedy a *vegetable mercury*. It's used for treatment of a sore throat that's worse on the right side, and also for treatment of mastitis.

51. *Pulsatilla nigricans* (wind flower). This remedy is a polychrest that's especially useful in the treatment of children; historically *Pulsatilla* has been described as a "female" remedy, as the emotional state is characterized by tearfulness and a need to be held and hugged. Complaints that fit this picture are improved by fresh air and worsened by heat. Children who need *Pulsatilla* are not thirsty, even if they have a high fever.

52. *Rhus toxicondenron* (poison ivy). This is a very important polychrest that's used for the treatment of poison ivy and poison oak. A professional homeopath might also find it useful for many different ailments, including obsessive-compulsive disorder (OCD). *Rhus* is well known for soothing arthritis when pain feels worse at the beginning of movement and improves as the person continues to move.

53. *Rumex crispus* (yellow dock). Tremendously important as a cough remedy, *Rumex* can help when a cough is worsened by changes of temperature (both from cold to warm and from warm to cold, as can happen when going in and out of climate-controlled buildings), as well as by taking a deep breath, talking, laughing, and uncovering. This cough is also made worse by pressure on the neck, including from bending the head forward. Compare this remedy with *Spongia*.

54. *Ruta graveolens* (garden rue). A remedy with many uses, *Ruta* helps treat injuries to tendons.

55. *Sabadilla officinalis* (cevadilla seed). *Sabadilla* is one of the main remedies for hay fever, especially when a person sneezes non-stop like a machine gun.

56. *Sambucus nigra* (elderberry). This is a very useful remedy for newborns with sniffles that prevent them from nursing. It's also very helpful for asthma when a child wakes up in the middle of the night with a feeling of suffocation. It can be also helpful in some cases of croup, whopping cough, and bronchitis.

57. *Spongia tosta* (roasted sponge). This remedy is one of the three most important remedies for croup (the others are *Aconitum* and *Hepar sulphur*). It's good for treating a dry, barking cough that might be described as sounding like "a saw going through wood." This cough is made better by warm drinks or food, and it's made worse by bending the head backward. Compare this remedy with *Rumex*.

58. *Stramonium* (thorn apple). This remedy is prescribed more frequently now, due to its significant effect on people who've gone through traumatic experiences, such as terrorist attacks and natural disasters. It's also indicated for children who often have vivid night-mares and develop other severe fears. We can thank renowned Greek homeopath George Vithoulkas for discovering the benefit of this remedy for these psychological conditions and prominent American homeopath Paul Herscu for writing his very good book, *Stramonium*, in which he further describes its characteristics. Unfortunately, the realities of the modern world are such that I must advise you to carry *Aconitum*, *Arnica*, and *Stramonium* in case of trauma.

59. *Sulphur* (brimstone). *Sulphur* is another polychrest, which is indicated for a child who is usually very warm—both physically and emotionally—and has a large appetite and a huge thirst for cold drinks.

60. *Symphytum officionale* (comfrey). This remedy is very use-ful in cases of broken bones. It helps fractures heal fast and strong.

61. *Tabacum* (tobacco). This remedy is useful for cases of severe car sickness and seasickness. Typically, the people who need it feel as though they will die from nausea. They become pale, almost green, cold, and sweaty. Their condition is much improved by cool air.

62. *Urtica urens* (stinging nettle). Practically a specific for allergic reactions to shellfish, this remedy is also helpful in treating burns and insect bites when the main complaint is a feeling of stinging and burning. In addition, *Urtica* helps women whose milk dries up too soon. A nice little remedy!

63. *Veratrum album* (white hellebore). Many physical and psychological conditions can be managed with this remedy. It is particularly useful for situations in which there's a combination of vomiting and diarrhea. As you might expect, children who benefit from this remedy can become very weak as a result of dehydration.

In Chapter Six, you'll learn about using specific remedies for acute conditions.

Chapter Six

Specific Remedies for Acute Conditions

In Chapter Five, you were introduced to sixty-three remedies that can form the basis of a remedy kit covering many of the most common acute ailments that crop up in the lives of pregnant and nursing women, infants, and growing children of all ages. With this special kit in hand, you'll be prepared to handle most of the acute conditions and emergency situations you could face in your home.

Here we'll explore a variety of acute conditions, their characteristics, and the specific remedies contained in your home kit that you should consider first when these conditions crop up. As you initially read this information, please hold in mind an essential principle of homeopathic prescribing: homeopathy treats individuals rather than diseases. Although this chapter is organized around the names of conditions, the remedies listed to treat them truly are only *potential* solutions.

Perhaps one day, this section of the book will become dog-eared from your having flipped through the pages so often. I imagine this book sitting on your bedside table. Please, before you begin using it like that, make sure to familiarize yourself with the contents of Chapter Seven, "Instructions for Using Homeopathic Remedies."

Dosing Instructions

Unless otherwise specified in the text, a homeopathic remedy should be given in the dose 30C, three pellets at a time. Three pellets are sufficient to cause a healing effect. If the instructions on the container are different than what I tell you in this book, please ignore them and follow the directions I have given. Please also be sure to read the section called "Choosing the Right Homeopathic Remedy for Your Child" in Chapter Seven.

After giving your child an initial dose of the remedy, wait for fifteen minutes, and evaluate your child's condition. If there is full improvement or the child goes to sleep, do not repeat the remedy. If you see no improvement, also do not repeat the remedy. However, if you see partial improvement, or if your child wakes up with the same complaint, give one more dose of the remedy. In severe conditions, if the first dose causes only partial improvement, repeating twice or even three times is OK.

Homeopathy for Pregnant and Nursing Mothers

Infants depend on their mothers in many different ways. First, they inherit their mother's emotional and physical traits. They're housed in the womb for about nine months, a location where they're subject to the same influences and experiences that the "housing authority" goes through during that time period. Then they're born. After birth, many babies are breast-fed by their mothers, which is how they receive essential nutrients and immune protection. If they are bottle-fed, this is not the case.

Of course, fathers also play an important role in their baby's life, but they're significantly more separated from babies than mothers are due to their biology.

As a mom, you need to be healthy. Homeopathy can help. It has been proven safe and efficacious in treating many of the ailments that pregnant and nursing women experience, including morning sickness, varicose veins, hemorrhoids, complications of labor, and sore nipples. Because homeopathic treatments have no side effects, you can only get stronger by using them. By extension, homeopathy will also be advantageous for your newborn.

In the initial section of the chapter, we'll talk about a few things you can do on your own during pregnancy, delivery, and breast-feeding to make events run smoothly.

Always contact your ob-gyn to consult on questionable situations, in addition to a homeopath. Your team of doctors provides a safety blanket for you and your baby.

Pregnancy

All of the mild complications of pregnancy can be managed beautifully with professional homeopathic treatment. There are some situations where you may be able to help yourself, too. For instance, you can easily navigate simple colds and flu during pregnancy by using the same strategies that we'll suggest for children later in the chapter. The remedies are identical and the results will be equally impressive.

Of course, it's always advisable to communicate even simple problems to your ob-gyn or midwife when you're pregnant. It's important to ensure that your acute condition won't complicate the course of pregnancy and the development of your baby.

When a problem of any kind—either an emotional one or a physical one—persists for more than a few days, you should seek professional help, as this might indicate a more serious problem. Consult a homeopathic doctor, if you can, and also get in touch with your ob-gyn. Do so expeditiously!

Morning Sickness

Conventional physicians often dismiss this condition as "natural" and suggest that pregnant women simply learn to live with it. But there are actually some natural home remedies to alleviate it. For instance, consuming preparations of ginger can help to a degree. Intensity of the nausea and vomiting can be so severe, however, that they not only cause extreme discomfort but also cause significant dehydration and weight loss. In these situations, morning sickness may become life threatening and require hospitalization.

In many cases, homeopathy provides safe and efficacious relief from morning sickness. I've seen miraculous cures after a woman had taken a single dose of a remedy, and I've also seen situations that required persistent trials of a variety of single remedies (one at a time) until the problem was relieved. In general, cases can be helped rather quickly.

Most likely, you'll have to take more than one dose of your chosen remedy. For this purpose, use the plussing method described in Chapter Two, in the section called "The Plussing Method: How to Prepare Liquid Remedies." If you vomit regularly, take an additional dose after each episode. If you don't throw up, repeat the remedy each time your nausea feels about 20 percent worse. An effective remedy lengthens the duration between episodes, so the period of relief becomes longer and longer.

The following list consists of remedies that are frequently indicated and can be used safely. Other remedies exist, but only professionals should prescribe them.

- *Anacardium orientalis*. This remedy is highly indicated if you wake up retching (dry heaves) but feel much better as soon as you eat. Compare indications for this remedy with those of *Nux vomica*.

- *Cocculus indicus*. This remedy is appropriate for the type of nausea that's like car sickness or seasickness. Use it if the mere sight of moving objects causes you dizziness and nausea. This is also the case if there's loathing of food. Another indication is that your condition gets worse when rising from bed or due to any other motion. This picture is of a combination of nausea from motion, odors, and food.

- *Colchicum autumnale*. This remedy is appropriate if you are nauseated by even the thought of food and if your condition is made worse by the odor and sight of food.

- *Natrum phosphoricum* (sodium phosphate). For nonspecific nausea in pregnancy, you can try this remedy, which has been reported to be very effective. I haven't seen it indicated frequently in my own practice.

- *Nux vomica*. This remedy is likely to resolve your condition if you wake up miserable and cranky and suffer from retching (dry heaves), and then you feel somewhat better in the afternoon but start off the next morning in the exact same way. Unlike *Ana-cardium*, the *Nux vomica* picture doesn't include getting better from eating. Eating actually makes things worse. Warm drinks can be helpful, but cold drinks cause more retching. People who need this remedy are usually irritable, with a very short fuse. They're highly sensitive to noises, light, and other forms of sensory input. Imagine someone who stays up too late and drinks too much coffee and so is tired and irritable. They'd fit this picture.

- *Phosphorus*. If you're very thirsty for cold drinks but throw up soon after you've had a gulp of water, this is probably your remedy. Fortunately, when it's indicated, one dose usually resolves the issue. The classic descriptor for this picture is vomiting as soon as the drink gets warm in the stomach.

Here's a cautionary note: if the first dose you take of any of these remedies doesn't work—if it doesn't provide even slight relief—do not repeat the remedy. Most probably, the remedy is wrong, and in this case repetition could make the situation worse. Seek professional help, especially if your morning sickness interferes with food intake!

Visiting a homeopath is a good idea if a remedy that brings initial relief of your nausea subsequently stops working for you. Most probably, you need someone to take a more sophisticated look at your problems. Remember to contact your homeopath and your ob-gyn as soon as possible.

Varicose Veins

Many women suffer from painfully enlarged and bulging veins during pregnancy. Some cases are fairly mild. Other cases are severely disfiguring and create significant discomfort. Frequently, *Hamamelis virginiana* is indicated for this ailment. Take three pellets twice a day of 6C potency and also apply *Hamamelis* ointment topically to your areas of discomfort. If you feel no relief in a few days, stop taking the pellets and go see a homeopath. You may also want to consult an allopathic physician.

Hemorrhoids

Hemorrhoids are another common, painful complication of pregnancy. Temporary relief can be provided with the use of homeopathic suppositories. OTC products contain combinations of different remedies, and many companies provide products that contain similar ingredients. These suppositories are easy to find in most health food stores, and some people swear by them. Professional homeopathic treatment also does miracles for patients suffering from hemorrhoids.

Labor

This is the big moment, the culmination of your pregnancy. Despite any frightening stories of various complications that you might have heard or read about, it's important to understand that childbirth is a natural process that a woman's body is built to do, and the logical resolution of pregnancy. Rest assured, the overwhelming majority of healthy women deliver their babies without complications.

Certainly, modern obstetrics provides a very safe environment for both mothers and babies. Only fathers are left to suffer from various levels of anxiety and even panic. I remember clearly how I felt at the end of a busy night at the clinic where I worked in Moscow when I received a phone call from my mother informing me that my wife had just gone to the hospital to deliver our second baby. I turned so red that the nurses suggested taking my blood pressure. You can bet it was high! Luckily, the birth only lasted thirty or forty minutes, so I didn't have enough time for a full-blown stroke.

All you men out there, becoming fathers, I feel for you! If you have a tendency to feel anxious and are easily excited, make sure that you get homeopathic help for yourself before the estimated date of delivery. You could be in for a lot of worry.

Certainly, mothers not only bear the children but also bear all physical consequences of pregnancy and labor. Homeopathy can be helpful for all of these. I've read several popular homeopathic books on the subject of pregnancy and delivery, which make numerous suggestions on various homeopathic remedies. Here's the reality of it: you, and even less so your anxious (actually, just plain scared) husband, won't be able to figure out what remedy to take for what symptom you experience in the middle of labor.

If you're delivering in a hospital, no homeopathic remedies will be allowed. Actually, if you were having an epidural, now a very popular painkilling procedure, no clear symptoms would be present anyhow. But that's OK. A lot of women decide to have an epidural for good reasons—no pain, minimal discomfort, everybody is happy. You can still utilize the general hints that I give in the following discussion, but don't go further. Realistically, if you need homeopathic treatment, it can be provided after your discharge from the hospital. Ideally, you won't have any problems and will never need it.

If you've made the choice to have a natural delivery, please make sure that you have a homeopath on board. Many midwives know elements of homeopathy. In many cases, they can recommend a homeopath in your area. Others are accomplished homeopaths themselves.

• *Arnica montana.* Those of you who've ever delivered know how exhausted and bruised women can feel afterward. It's a good idea to take *Arnica* 200C as soon as the baby has emerged from your birth canal, as it's a great remedy for many of labor's consequences. As more physicians are becoming familiar with alternative medicine, you may want to discuss this ahead of time with your obstetrician so you'll have a clear understanding and won't need to hide anything. Midwives are more open-minded. The dose can be safely repeated in a few hours.

Arnica helps heal the incisions from an episiotomy. In the case of natural tearing, it may not be as helpful, but it most certainly isn't going to hurt. If you've previously given birth and believe that ineffective contractions won't be an issue for you, consider utilizing the *Arnica* protocol for surgery that's described in Chapter Five.

• *Caulophyllum thalictroides*. Some homeopaths call this remedy "*Arnica* for labor." A 200C dose, or even a 30C dose, taken at the beginning of labor may save you from trouble with painful, ineffective contractions. But the remedy can also be given at a later stage in labor.

In my experience, taking one dose is sufficient so long as the remedy is indicated initially by painful, ineffective contractions. Of course, if you plan to deliver in the hospital, you may want to take a dose prophylactically on your way there, as the experts I have mentioned suggest. Individualized treatment is always better than "cookie cutter" recommendations. Constitutional treatment during pregnancy and before labor usually provides a much better prognosis for smooth delivery.

• *Calendula officinalis* (marigold). An ointment or gel applied to a wound (after an episiotomy or a tear) helps ensure proper healing of the vaginal opening without inflammation. Taking a *Calendula* 12C pellet once daily for ten to fourteen days in combination with the application of the ointment or gel twice a day provides a very good environment for the wound healing.

• *Carbo vegetabilis*. This remedy performs miracles for women who feel exhausted during or after labor. The need to be fanned is a very important feature in its picture. Sometimes women ask for so much air from the fan or the air conditioner that everybody else in the room freezes. A dose in 200C or 30C can bring about a dramatic recovery of energy, and it helps women complete their job.

• *Staphysagria* (delphinium seed). In the case of painful tearing, an episiotomy that had to be performed, or a Caesarean section accompanied with feelings of emotional hurt and a sense of being humiliated, a dose of this remedy goes a long way. If you're in doubt, wait until you can consult with your homeopath. Taking the other remedies described earlier in this section beforehand won't interfere with the action of *Staphysagria* if it ultimately should be taken. Even so, sooner is always better.

Postpartum Bleeding (Uterine Hemorrhage)

Beware! Postpartum hemorrhage is a serious, potentially life-threatening problem. No time should be spared in getting professional help if it occurs. Excessive bleeding always has a serious underlying cause that needs to be investigated. Delaying emergency assistance could be dangerous, especially if surgery is required. Bleeding can occur during delivery or soon after delivery. It can also occur a week, or even more, following delivery.

Homeopathy can offer effective solutions for all of these types of bleeding, but the professional obstetric-gynecological evaluation must take place in a hospital setting. Most information on the homeopathic treatment of uterine bleeding was written in the days when there were homeopathic hospitals in the United States. These no longer exist. Therefore take note of the following:

- In the case of excessive bleeding during a home delivery, you should be on your way to the emergency room right away.
- In the case of excessive bleeding during a hospital birth, you'll be treated with allopathic medications, with no access to homeopathy allowed.
- When the bleeding occurs a week or even more after delivery, remedies shouldn't be administered without proper obstetrical evaluation.

I don't approve of the cavalier approach of some contemporary homeopathic authors who expect women (or their family members) to self-prescribe for this dangerous condition. I only decided to write about this issue to give you an additional warning about the necessity of promptly seeking professional help.

Postpartum Blues (Depression)

Often postpartum blues are transitory and last only for the few days immediately after delivery. But if you have this problem for more than a few days, please be aware that it can become extremely serious and may negatively affect you and your baby. Left without prompt treatment, it could require serious psychiatric intervention—and perhaps even hospitalization.

I've treated a significant number of women for postpartum depression with very good results. Homeopathy can do miracles for this condition. But, without a doubt, you must see an experienced homeopath to resolve this issue. Depressed people cannot make good decisions. Therefore self-treatment in this case isn't a good idea. In fact, treating complicated emotional problems on your own is never a good idea for either you or your children.

Breast-Feeding

Breast-feeding provides joy to both mother and baby. It also gives babies immune protection from infections and ensures better digestion and a healthier later life. Luckily, the majority of mothers understand it, and the latest fashion of bottle-feeding seems to be over. Of course, the process takes two to tango, and problems may arise on both sides.

Milk Production (Too Little). The majority of mothers have no problem producing a sufficient amount of milk to satisfy their baby's needs. The most common cause of insufficient milk is inadequate fluid intake by the mother. You can't make milk out of air. Women under constitutional homeopathic care usually fare well overall, breast-feeding included. Nonetheless some have this problem. Fortunately, quite a few remedies can be helpful.

As always, if you've had enough to drink and are still having a problem, it's best to get advice from a professional homeopath, and consider a lactation consultant, as well—they can be found through La Leche League. Changes in milk production can be indicative of a larger, systemic problem. If you have no access to a homeopath or must wait for an appointment, consider the following three remedies:

- *Ignatia amara.* This remedy is helpful in cases in which there's a direct correlation between the loss of milk and the emotional strain connected with having a new baby. If there's a connection like this, one dose of 200C should be sufficient to restore a mother's balance. Certainly, if the emotional strain is due to family discord, the situation has an apparent cause that also needs to be addressed. There is no "magic pill" for that type of issue.

- *Pulsatilla nigricans.* This is a very helpful remedy if you want to increase milk production. Emotional indicators, such as weepiness; changeable, irritable moods; or merely an increased need for attention and sympathy, can point you toward choosing this remedy.

A daily 30C dose for a few days usually brings about a result. You should stop taking the remedy if milk production goes up to the desired level or if there is no effect. Repeat the remedy only if you see some response after the first dose.

- *Castor oil.* If applied directly on the breast, it can help increase milk production. There is a homeopathic remedy *Ricinus communis* made from castor bean. I've never prescribed it and cannot recommend it for general use. Homeopaths—myself included—know the indications for this remedy well, and we'll be perfectly able to recommend it if you have the appropriate picture of symptoms.

Milk Production (Too Much). Some women suffer from excessive milk production. Interestingly, *Pulsatilla nigricans* can regulate and decrease milk production in women who have too much. In the event that there's a plan not to breast-feed, for whatever reason, *Pulsatilla* can be taken immediately after the birth of the baby—even before any characteristic symptoms develop. That usually halts milk production. In the opinion of some homeopaths, *Bryonia* can also be useful to halt production.

Cracked and Sore Nipples. For breast-feeding to be pleasant for mother and baby, a woman's nipples must be soft and without cracks. Sore, cracked nipples make breast-feeding difficult and painful, and they also present a high risk for development of a breast infection (mastitis).

One of the best substances for breast care is *Calendula officinalis* ointment or gel. Massaging the nipples with *Calendula* can prevent the occurrence of cracks and soreness. Castor oil is another great healer, even for advanced cases of cracked nipples. Ultimately, your personal preference should dictate which one you use. You might try alternating one with the other for a few days to see which works better.

Mastitis (Breast Infection). Frequently, if not always, breast infections result from plugged milk ducts. Some people refer to this condition as having a *caked breast*. The initial soreness caused by mastitis is usually relieved either by feeding an active, hungry baby or by active breast pumping. If the milk ducts don't unplug following these efforts and the infection is exacerbated, or if the reason for the infection is a cracked nipple, there's an excellent homeopathic remedy to treat mastitis, called *Phytolacca decandra*.

I have seen *Phytolacca* work in many cases of initial mastitis, and sometimes even in progressed cases. During our immigration from Russia, my wife, my daughters, and I were housed in Ladispoli, Italy. One of the families in our group had a very young child whose breast-feeding mother had to attend many different interviews and apparently hadn't pumped too well beforehand. As a result, she developed a severe case of mastitis, with breast tenderness, redness, pain, and fever. The problem emerged during the weekend, when there was no access to medical care.

I had *Phytolacca* 6X in my bags and offered it to the woman. Remedies at this concentration have to be taken at least three times a day. In less than twenty-four hours, the swelling and tenderness went down, and in another day the episode was over. Homeopathy works well even under the most difficult conditions.

Normally, I recommend taking one 30C dose and then—if you've seen an initial positive effect after that first dose—switching to the plussing method (see Chapter Two). Continue taking the liquid preparation every three to four hours until resolution of the problem.

Do not stop the breast-feeding. The only reasonable excuse not to breast-feed your child is having a severe contagious infection, such as AIDS or tuberculosis. Of course, there may be other infections to consider. When in doubt, consult your primary care provider. All other ailments, including the flu, shouldn't affect your feeding schedule. Of course, you should follow all hygienic advice, including the application of oils after rinsing the nipples to keep them soft. You should also read the section later in this chapter on homeopathic treatment of colds and flu. Frequently, if *Phytolacca* doesn't work right away, one of the remedies for colds may be indicated, remedies such as *Belladonna, Bryonia,* or *Eupatorium.*

If there's no improvement within twenty-four hours of your first attempt to address this problem, you should consult a homeopath. If that's impossible, consult an allopathic physician. This issue has to be resolved efficiently and quickly with the involvement of professionals on every level of care as necessary. If you develop recurrent mastitis, homeopathic consultation is highly indicated.

Sniffles in Newborns

When an infant cannot nurse, you're facing a very unfortunate occurrence. There are many steps you can take before turning to homeopathic treatment, but if an infant's nasal obstruction becomes so pronounced that the child can't nurse, use *Sambucus* 30C. You can dilute the pellet in a small amount of water (let's say two tablespoons), or in your own breast milk if the baby refuses to drink water. Then stir or shake the preparation vigorously and give the child half a teaspoon of it. You can repeat the dose one more time in thirty minutes if the improvement is only partial. Don't do anything else unless you see a significant improvement. If there is no effect at all, immediately consult your physician. Your baby must be able to breast-feed and receive nourishment.

Milk Intolerance in Babies

Mother's milk is the best food for an infant. However, some babies reject it. If this happens, first of all, you should make sure that your emotional-physical condition is as good as it can be. In some cases, what you're eating can make the milk taste unpleasant. In any case, if rejection occurs or if the baby vomits breast milk frequently, you should consult your physician. If everything turns out to be OK with you and the baby, but the baby still refuses your milk or vomits your milk, consult a homeopath.

There is a great homeopathic remedy for babies who vomit milk frequently, *Aethusa cynapium* 30C.

Treating Acute Conditions with Homeopathy

Unlike the majority of homeopathic self-help books on the market, this book only teaches you how to help your child with self-limiting, easy-to-recognize, and easy-to-treat conditions. You don't need to become a doctor. Do your best in selecting a remedy, and in most cases, your child will recover quickly. But if your child doesn't improve in fifteen to thirty minutes, don't panic, and don't keep on trying different remedies, hoping that one of them will ultimately get the job done. Instead follow up with a professional homeopath (or an allopathic physician). Remember, better safe than sorry!

Accidents and Emergencies—Homeopathic First Aid

Internally taken remedies are much more effective than external applications, such as ointments and gels, although you're certainly welcome to use both kinds of remedies in serious cases. Please remember, there's no need to treat every single fall or bruise with an internal remedy. Minor conditions like bumps and bruises may be treated with ointments—or with a kiss and a hug. But serious injuries and traumas require that you take quick, decisive action. In such situations, don't waste any time! Give your child a remedy and call 9-1-1. Or give the remedy and go to the nearest ER.

In cases of significant trauma, feel free to repeat the remedy every fifteen minutes, as long as there are signs of improvement. You should stop when the improvement plateaus.

- *Arnica montana* is the most important remedy to have for trauma. In situations when you have nothing else available, *Arnica* will always provide some degree of help to a traumatized child. It's an excellent remedy for a baby who has gone through a stressful birth, like a forceps delivery, a breech birth, or prolonged labor. It also does wonders in cases of extremely severe trauma, such as natural disasters, industrial accidents, or automobile accidents. Ever since witnessing a terrible motorcycle accident right in front of me on the highway, I have kept a container of *Arnica* 10M in the glove compartment of my car. *Arnica* is amazing!

A famous homeopathic couple, Roger Morrison and Nancy Herric, happened to be on Bali during a terrorist attack that happened in October 2002. Roger is an experienced ER doctor and Nancy is a physician's assistant, so they volunteered in the local hospital. They had only a handful of remedies. Roger told me that *Arnica* performed miracles.

The more severe the trauma you're confronting, the higher the potency should be. Often 200C is appropriate. If there's an initial effect, you should then repeat the dose until you reach the plateau of improvement.

Very characteristic symptoms are the following:

- Experiencing initial shock: the person feels OK and refuses help despite severe injuries.
- Having significant soreness, feeling beaten, or the bed seems too hard.
- Developing a nosebleed after trauma to a different area or while washing the face or coughing. Famous American homeopath Paul Herscu has described a case in which a pregnant woman developed uterine bleeding after washing her face. Her pregnancy was saved by a single dose of *Arnica*.

Here's a cautionary note: never apply *Arnica* ointment, or another external *Arnica* preparation, on broken skin, as it will cause severe irritation.

Other remedies that may be indicated for blunt trauma include the following:

• *Aconitum napellus*. Select this remedy if feelings of great terror dominate all other symptoms. It's usually indicated in the first moments after a horrific trauma.

• *Bellis perenis*. Use this remedy if there's been trauma to internal organs, such as the liver, spleen, or uterus. It's also appropriate if much swelling remains for a long time after an injury such as a sprain, despite administering *Arnica* or any other appropriate remedy.

• *Bryonia alba*. This remedy is appropriate if even the slightest motion hurts, and if the victim absolutely refuses to move. The condition is made better from firm pressure, and from lying on the injured part of the body. Please note that you should seriously consider this remedy each time trauma to the bones is involved.

• *Carbo vegetabilis*. The main indications for this remedy are that shock following severe injury is characterized by severe weakness and significant coldness of the injured area. The victim faints and needs constant fanning.

• *Hamamelis virginiana*. This remedy is useful for severe bruises that swell and bleed. It's also useful for nosebleeds that last a long time, even after you give *Arnica*. It's a specific remedy for traumatic bleeding inside the eye.

• *Hypericum perforatum*. This remedy is appropriate for crushing injuries to fingers and toes.

• *Ledum palustre*. This remedy is appropriate for puncture wounds, including insect stings.

• *Ruta graveolens*. Use this remedy for trauma to the periosteum, or connective tissue that wraps around the bones, especially in areas where the bone is close to the skin, like the shinbone, the pelvis, and the elbow.

Asthma Attack

Asthma is an emergency, and it has to be treated as such, with a 9-1-1 response triggered as soon as necessary. Treatment of asthma is complicated. I've seen amazing results with constitutional homeopathic treatment of chronic cases and even more amazing results with homeopathic treatment of acute attacks. You shouldn't attempt to serve as your child's doctor. A physician should handle this emergency. Ideally, consult a homeopath for constitutional care and create an emergency plan with remedy choices in the event of an acute attack.

While you're waiting for professional help, consider a few remedies (obviously, there are many more possibilities). I will list them in the order of usefulness. Give your child the remedy in potency 30C, and repeat if the improvement that follows is only partial or if the symptoms begin to come back. With each new dose, if your child doesn't reach the same level of improvement as with the previous dose, the remedy is wrong and you should stop. The best-case scenario is that professional help is already on its way.

- *Sambucus.* A child wakes up in the middle of the night frightened by suffocation. Indications include a cough and a blue face. This often happens in connection with acute bronchitis or sinusitis. Usually, the child also presents with profuse perspiration right after waking up from the asthma attack. *Sambucus* is a very frequently indicated remedy.
- *Antimonium tartaricum.* This remedy is usually appropriate if the asthma attack is a result of infection. Think about this remedy first if a child has a lot of mucus in the chest that rattles on breathing in and breathing out. Nothing comes out during cough. But when the child finally emits a small amount of very sticky yellow mucus, breathing becomes markedly better. The child is usually irritable and wants to be left alone.

- *Apis mellifica*. This remedy is used for allergic asthma that's associated with hives and swelling of the face, lips, and neck. Breathing is very tight and painful.
- *Arsenicum album*. This is indicated for asthma attacks due to either allergy or infection. The child is frequently worse between midnight and 2 A.M. The child cannot lie down but must sit up or even bend forward. The child is very *anxious, restless,* and *fearful* and also thirsty for sips of cold drinks. If you see a case of asthma when the child gets better after lying down at night, give *Euphrasia officinalis*.
- *Ipecacuanha*. This remedy is useful when there's a constant cough with gagging and vomiting.

Bites and Insect Stings

Please remember that most often stings and insect bites don't require any kind of treatment. Parents frequently overuse homeopathic remedies in cases of minor falls and insect bites, even though an uncomplicated sting from one bee doesn't require a remedy. My favorite external application for bee stings is Gold Star balm, which is sold in Chinese and Korean stores. It comes in a cute little red tin container with, as you might imagine, a gold star on it. A single application usually takes the itching and stinging feeling away and also reduces local swelling. Ssstingstop™, a combination homeopathic topical gel can also work wonders. If you don't have a balm handy, ice and a little bit of aloe vera would probably solve the problem.

If your child has a systemic reaction to an insect bite or a sting, or if the area becomes significantly swollen and very painful, a homeopathic remedy does miracles.

Animal and human bites present significant problems, as they get quickly infected and have a tendency to heal slowly with a lot of complications. Homeopathic remedies promote faster healing and decrease or sometimes even prevent scar formation. The sooner you give the remedy, the better the outcome will be. Please don't forget to clean the wound, too. Hydrogen peroxide is always a good choice, because it kills many types of dangerous bacteria and also cleans the wound very well.

The following are remedies that are useful in treating stings and bites:

- *Aconitum napellus*. I've seen cases when a child stung by a bee gets so scared that the need for *Aconitum* is obvious. Use it if your child is scared, red faced, and has an expression of terror such that the pupils of the eyes become very small. One dose of *Aconitum* 30C will resolve this issue, and then you have to wait and see. Taking this remedy may be sufficient, or the child may also develop symptoms afterward that indicate a need for another remedy listed in the following discussion.

- *Apis mellifica*. Use this remedy if the area of a sting is swollen red, warm to the touch, and the condition is made better by cold. (Compare with the picture of *Ledum* in which the area is usually cold and reddish blue.) Frequently, the child who needs *Apis* is quite irritable; it's easy for the child to fly off the handle.

I've seen cases of severe allergic reactions to bee stings that almost instantly respond to *Apis*. Severe swelling with inflammation after stings from other insects responds similarly well. A dose of 30C is good, either dry or in water (for example, the plussing method). If there's an initial, but not a complete, improvement, repeat the dose two more times at thirty- to sixty-minute intervals. Stop giving doses sooner if the child is more than 50 percent better.

Don't use *Apis*, or any other remedy for that matter, just because there's a situation in which it's frequently indicated. Frequently, the bites of wasps and other large insects require *Ledum*— but not always. Assess what's going on with your child for a few minutes before making your selection.

- *Ledum palustre*. This remedy is almost a specific for animal bites (including those from dogs, cats, raccoons, and snakes) and human bites, and for the stings and bites of large insects, such as wasps. A main indication is that the area of the bite or sting is reddish blue and surrounded by a very pale area. The wound is also cold to the touch. (Compare with *Apis*.)

Paradoxically, ice-cold applications bring about a dramatic improvement although the areas of the bite are cold. In this picture, the child won't let go of the ice pack! (Compare with the picture of *Arsenicum* in which the area is hot, and the pain is improved by hot applications. If that happens and your child is anxious, *Arsenicum* should be your first choice.)

• *Urtica urens*. This remedy is used for stings of jellyfish and medusa. It's also used for any other type of insect bites or stings in which the main symptoms are hives and itching that get better from rubbing the area. Some children start rubbing the wound nonstop.

Homeopathy is effective in the treatment of bites by scorpions, snakes, and spiders. It's also effective for treatment of severe allergic reactions to bites and stings, including anaphylactic shock (a severe allergic reaction that is sometimes fatal). From the following list, please find a description of a few remedies that can be helpful with these issues. If you're an avid traveler and your family spends time in the wilderness, make sure you have these remedies handy, along with other first aid items.

• *Carbolicum acidum*. This is a remedy of choice for severe allergic reactions to bee stings, insect bites, and animal bites. It's also very useful for anaphylaxis. In this picture, a child has a dusky red face, but the skin around the mouth and nose is pale. The victim also reports a choking feeling and frequently becomes lethargic but even so may paradoxically develop an acute awareness of odors. In cases of allergic reactions, a child develops hives over the entire body.

Give repeated 30C doses every ten to fifteen minutes until improvement or the arrival of the ambulance. You should *always* call 9-1-1 or go to the ER if you see these symptoms develop. If the condition arises during your camping trip, give the remedy and head toward a populated area as fast as you can!

• *Lachesis muta.* Constantine Hering discovered this major homeopathic polychrest over a hundred years ago. In cases of poisonous bites by snakes or spiders, it can be beneficial. The affected part has a dusky, purple color. Frequently, you'll see a continuous oozing of blood from the wound.

Give a 200C dose once and apply an ice pack to prevent the poison from spreading. Of course, professional help *must* be on its way, or you should be rushing toward the nearest hospital right away!

• *Oxalicum acidum.* This remedy works very well if the affected part becomes numb and cold to the touch, and the victim also reports violent pains and begins to tremble. It's imperative to rush the victim to the nearest hospital! Give one dose of the remedy on your way.

Burns

Serious burns always have to be treated in a hospital setting. You shouldn't delay seeking professional medical attention. Rush the burn victim to the hospital and give the best remedy you can on the route there.

For minor burns, Hahnemann advised using warm applications, a practice that makes sense homeopathically. A more radical technique exists that originated in folk medicine: an application (preferably direct) of the victim's own fresh urine is advised after the minor burn. I've witnessed the amazing effect of this seemingly strange method on many injured people and have even experienced it firsthand. It works miracles for minor incidents like being scalded with spilled hot tea or coffee. Of course, the majority of burn victims ask to be given cold applications. Folk medicine also recommends touching your own earlobe in cases of minor burns to the fingertips, as the earlobe is usually cold.

After cleaning the burned area and making sure it's dry, apply *Calendula* ointment or lotion. Then give one of these remedies if the picture seems appropriate.

- *Apis mellifica*. Use this remedy for a minor burn that's greatly relieved by ice-cold applications and is red and swollen. It's also helpful for chemical burns to the eyes. Here's a note of caution: if you don't know how to handle chemical burns, don't interfere with the efforts of trained professionals or a first-response team.
- *Arsenicum album*. This remedy is beneficial for severe burns (third degree), and for burns accompanied by significant anxiety and restlessness. Note that the victim refuses cold applications and feels better from warm applications.
- *Cantharis*. This is usually used for second-degree and third-degree burns with extreme burning pain (remember how the sting of nettles feels). Unlike the victim's response that indicates *Arsenicum*, this victim desires ice-cold applications. The patient simply wouldn't let go of an ice pack. It works for chemical burns, too. It's important to note that a prompt administration of this remedy may prevent the formation of blisters.
- *Urtica urens*. Urtica is beneficial for minor burns caused by scalding-hot boiling water.

Furthermore, if your child is terrified by the traumatic experience of being burned, *Aconitum napellus* is appropriate.

Concussions

Injuries to the head cannot be treated lightly. You always need to make sure that the victim receives a full neurological workup that includes brain-imaging studies. On the way to the emergency room, consider the following remedies:

- *Aconitum napellus*. Aconitum is very useful when dealing with fright and terror, and often a full-blown fear of death, in the first moments after the head injury.

• *Arnica montana*. *Arnica* is the most frequently indicated remedy for a banged head. A victim often denies having a problem and refuses an examination. In fact, I've witnessed this symptom on numerous occasions, even when one homeopath was injured in front of several other homeopaths. In this particular case, everyone was concerned except him. That's why the analysis of the case took literally only a few seconds. *Arnica* saved this man from severe complications. Another possible scenario is that a victim goes in and out of a stupor, kind of falling asleep and waking up again. In this picture, you'll frequently notice significant bruising.

• *Ferrum phosphoricum*. If you see signs of fever after head injury, think of *Ferrum*. A dose of this remedy can make a dramatic difference in such cases. Allopathic physicians don't have a specific medication for this condition.

Many other remedies are especially helpful for chronic changes after a head injury. Treatment of these consequences, even the most severe ones, can be very successful. In severe cases, that treatment should be managed by an experienced homeopath.

Croup

Croup can be a scary situation, as a child may develop significant difficulty in breathing relatively quickly. Homeopathy handles this problem very well. A correct remedy aborts the development of further complications and quickly reverses the illness. But don't waste any time. Give the best remedy you can pick, and if the child isn't better in ten to fifteen minutes, or if breathing is extremely labored from the beginning, call 9-1-1 or go to the ER. Give the remedy as you're on your way to the hospital.

• *Aconitum napellus*. *Aconitum* is the most important remedy in the beginning of the illness. I know firsthand of many cases when a single dose at the onset of croup symptoms swiftly cured a child. The child wakes up with a dry (no mucus!), barking, suffocating cough. The child is scared and clings to parents. Breathing gets worse with every breath.

Give a 30C dose and call 9-1-1. Remember, when *Aconitum* is indicated, no mucus is present. If there's mucus, the child needs a different remedy.

- *Spongia tosta.* Another important and commonly needed remedy is *Spongia*. In this picture, the child has a dry, barking cough, with the sound frequently described as "a saw going through wood" or "like a seal's bark." The child may wake up scared. The condition is made better by nursing, eating, or drinking, and from bending the head forward. (Compare with *Hepar sulphur.*)

- *Hepar sulphur.* Croup often develops between 2 A.M. and 4 A.M., or even later. There is thick, rattling mucus. The child might get much worse from uncovering even a small part of the body and cannot tolerate anything cold. Frequently, the child is irritable and touchy. With this symptom, the child feels better from throwing the head backward. (Compare with *Spongia.*)

- *Sambucus.* *Sambucus* is indicated less frequently than the previously listed remedies. A very specific symptom is waking up with profuse perspiration that accompanies the cough and breathing difficulties.

Dental Work

Many children find the experience of dental work emotionally or physically traumatic and sometimes both. Homeopathy can help.

- *Aconitum napellus.* One dose of *Aconitum* can dramatically transform the emotional state of a child who's morbidly terrified of dental work. In this picture, children may feel that they'll die from having a dental procedure. You can give one dose of 30C right before leaving the house and another dose, if your child is still fearful, on arrival at the dentist's office. There are numerous remedies for fearful, anxious children. If these are ongoing problems, make an appointment with a homeopath.

- *Arnica montana.* This is an excellent remedy for the treat-ment of pain, bleeding, and other complications arising after den-tal surgery and tooth extraction. Let's take the example of my older daughter, who had four wisdom teeth removed in one session at age seventeen. All of her classmates told her that she'd be out of school for a week, suffering from terrible pain and swelling. The dentist prescribed an antibiotic for her that he wanted her to begin taking prophylactically before the surgery and for a few days after. We decided to hold off and see if it was needed.

I instructed my wife, who was taking our daughter to the den-tist's office, to give our daughter *Arnica* 200C immediately after the surgery was over. As you know, local anesthesia makes your mouth numb. Therefore somebody has to put the pellet in the mouth for the recipient. It doesn't have to go under the tongue. Placing a pel-let or two between the lower lip and the gum is fine. The dentist prescribed three different painkillers to be taken around the clock. My daughter took the dose of whatever he wanted her to take in the office. An hour later, I gave her another dose of *Arnica* 200C. That same day, she had a few friends over and was talking, laugh-ing, and eating without any problems—no bleeding, no pain, no infection. We never gave her the antibiotic.

I gave one more dose of *Arnica* that first night and that was it. Certainly, we had a supply of the antibiotic that the dentist had recommended, and my wife bought two out of the three painkillers that the dentist had prescribed, even though our daughter didn't end up needing them.

My dentist knows about the power of *Arnica* and places a pel-let that I bring to my own dental surgery appointments in my mouth immediately after he's done. He wears surgical gloves and is allowed to touch the pill. *Arnica* is just amazing!

- *Chamomilla.* This remedy is indicated for children (and adults) who are extremely sensitive to pain, including dental pain. This type of child will make various arrangements with the dentist to signal even the slightest pain. Any procedure becomes a night-mare for both the patient and the doctor. Instead of giving Valium to the dentist (just kidding), you might want to try giving the child *Chamomilla* 30C before the procedure.

- *Gelsemium sempervirens*. Use this remedy if a child is very anxious, fearful, and weak. It's especially appropriate if there's great weakness after the procedure and the child trembles upon rising. The *Gelsemium* state includes an anxiety that's similar to stage fright, rather than terror or panic to the point of fearing death, as in the state of *Aconitum*.

Drowning

If someone has been rescued from drowning, the most important things to do are to act calmly, call 9-1-1, assign someone to clear the area of spectators, and start performing cardiopulmonary resuscitation (CPR). If you don't know how to do CPR, ask around. Usually, someone in every crowd is trained in CPR for victims of near drowning.

The remedy of choice under these circumstances is *Antimonium tartaricum* 30C. Give a pellet to the unconscious person as soon as you can. But be sure to moisten the pellet with water first, and then carefully place it between the cheek and the gum, so the victim doesn't choke on it. Repeat the dose three times at ten- to fifteen-minute intervals. Stop when the victim is conscious and breathing, even if it happens after the first dose.

Remember to call 9-1-1 right away, before you do anything else. If you're busy attending to the victim, delegate someone else to do it ASAP!

Eye Injuries

First of all, if there is a speck in the eye, it needs to be removed by flushing out. Never touch the eye with anything dry! To relieve any irritation and pain after the removal of a foreign body in the eye, add half a teaspoon of *Calendula* tincture to a cup of cold water, and then use this mixture as an eyewash. You can also use it to flush out the speck. And remember, we live in twenty-first-century United States of America! An eye doctor is always available! So go to the doctor.

The following remedies are useful in cases of eye injuries:

* *Aconitum napellus.* Old-time homeopaths used to call this remedy "*Arnica* of the eye." It relives pain and inflammation. Remember, you might get temporary relief even if the speck is still in the eye, but the pain will ultimately come back until it's removed. Sometimes children will not allow you even to open their eyes. Give *Aconitum* and bring them to the eye doctor or the ER.
* *Arnica montana.* This remedy is useful for a black eye caused by walking into a door, or by receiving a blow above or below the eye.
* *Calendula officinalis.* To treat bleeding for a cut eyelid, soak a gauze pad in a mixture of half a teaspoon of *Calendula* tincture and a cup of cold water, and then apply the pad to the cut with gentle pressure.
* *Hypericum perforatum.* Give one dose of 30C internally for severe pain in the eye after the injury. You can also prepare an eyewash from *Hypericum* tincture (use similar proportions to *Calendula*) and use it externally.
* *Ledum palustre. Ledum* is beneficial for a black eye that feels much better from cold applications.
* *Symphytum officinalis. Symphytum* is used for injury directly to the eyeball.

Fever

Most of us know that fever is a good thing, as it provides a better environment for our immune system to function and a much worse environment for the microbes. Fever is not an illness. It's a symptom that signals that there's a problem—most probably an infection—and that our body is beginning to fight it. Suppressing a fever is similar to saying, "Just shut up!" to someone warning you of enemies coming to your house.

Homeopathy addresses the core issue. That's why we choose the remedy for fever based on the person's whole presentation. Homeopathic remedies are perfectly capable of halting the development of any infection, and they help to restore total health. The effect is very quick. If you don't see any improvement in thirty minutes after giving a remedy, seek professional help. Very high fevers can be dangerous. If your child's fever goes down, but new symptoms come up, the remedy you gave was good, but not perfect, and you also need to consult a doctor. Give one dose of 30C and wait for fifteen to twenty minutes. Frequently, the child feels much better and goes to sleep. If there is a flare-up of the fever with the same picture of core symptoms, repeat the remedy.

By the way, don't automatically give repeated doses every fifteen minutes. That isn't going to speed up recovery. Here I've only listed remedies that are frequently indicated. In some cases, treatment of fevers can be tricky.

- *Aconitum napellus*. Use if the onset is very sudden, as frequently happens after a child is exposed to cold wind. Often significant chills precede this fever, and the child's temperature usually rises in the evening or at night. The child is very thirsty and the pupils are small. (Compare with *Belladonna*.)

These mental symptoms indicate using *Aconitum*: excitement with fear and restlessness. If the child isn't excited and restless, *Aconitum* probably isn't a good choice. Physical symptoms that suggest using *Aconitum*: thirsty for cold, may have one cheek red, another pale (similar to *Chamomilla*).

- *Arsenicum album*. In this state, the child is restless, but it's unlike the *Aconitum* state. It isn't from terror. It's from significant anxiety. The child complains of burning pains (for example, in the throat), which are made better by warm applications. *Burning better from warmth* is a symptom that's unique to this remedy. The child is also thirsty for cold water, but only in small sips. (Compare with *Aconitum*, *Bryonia*, and *Phosphorus* states, in which the child has a thirst for large amounts of cold water.) The face is hot; the rest of the body is cold. Head symptoms are better from cold, symptoms in the rest of the body from heat.

• *Belladonna*. This remedy is probably the most frequently prescribed homeopathic remedy for fever. The picture is usually very clear. The child may be confused. It does not always happen all the time, but the child often looks somewhat "off." Eyes are glassy. Pupils are large. (Compare with *Aconitum*.) In some cases, you may notice slight twitching of the face and the body or even febrile seizures. The face and body are hot to the touch, and the hands and feet are cold. (Don't get stuck on this last symptom. If it's there, go for it. If not, look at everything else.)

The child has no thirst or specifically asks for lemonade or lemons. Sometimes the child initially has chills. These usually occur in the afternoon and begin in the arms or in the abdomen.

• *Bryonia alba*. Fever usually develops slowly. Interestingly, the chills (if they happen) begin either at 9 A.M. or 9 P.M. and start in the fingertips, toes, or lips. Children in this state complain of pains and want to be *absolutely still, quiet, left alone*. They may become confused, then they are characteristically scared that they aren't at home and ask to go home. They have an incredible thirst for large amounts of very cold water; they cannot have enough. When chilly, the face is white. When the fever rises, the face becomes deep red.

• *Chamomilla*. This remedy is very useful in treating small children, especially during dentition. A combination of new teeth coming out, fever, irritability, and capriciousness should red flag it for you. Additional signs are that the child calms down only if carried in someone's arms, and sometimes you can see that one cheek is red and the other pale. Combined with other symptoms, this last indicator confirms your choice. It's also a good remedy for situations when a high fever doesn't come down for a long time. The heat is frequently intolerable.

• *Ferrum phosphoricum*. This is an important remedy. But people have a tendency either to ignore it or to overuse it. Overuse comes from its leading characteristic: *no specific symptoms*. Indeed children who need this remedy don't develop any local symptoms or any significant general unique symptoms. Yes, their face may be red, and they may have a sore throat or an earache, but there's nothing distinctive about these symptoms. A mistake is made when parents rush to give *Ferrum* right away, without carefully looking into what's going on. However, if you wait for a few hours after your child becomes feverish and you still don't see anything specific, give a dose of this remedy. You could get excellent results.

The onset of a condition that needs *Ferrum* is usually gradual. The child may look as if *Belladonna* is needed, but there's no confusion and the symptoms are milder. Many old-time books suggest that girls commonly need this remedy. The better way to understand it is that the reaction is mild, not dramatic. Still, the child might have a headache and feel better from cold compresses to the head.

• *Gelsemium sempervirens*. *Gelsemium* is indicated for fever accompanied by tremendous weakness. The child can be trembling from weakness and sometimes cannot even open the eyes. Chills are running up and down the child's back, and the back of the head feels very heavy. Often there's an occipital headache. The child may have blurry vision and at times even double vision. The limbs are also heavy. Amazingly, despite having a high fever, the child is not thirsty.

• *Phosphorus*. You should think about this remedy if a child with a high fever (103 to 104 degrees) remains active and appears perfectly well. The child is also thirsty for cold drinks, is chilly, has night sweats, and has a cold moving into the chest.

Fainting

The following three remedies are appropriate when dealing with fainting:

• *Carbo vegetabilis*. This remedy is appropriate when a child requires constant fanning. The condition is much improved from fresh air.

- *Chamomilla*. This is indicated for fainting from severe pain.
- *Coffea cruda*. This is a remedy appropriate for fainting from excitement.

While often benign, fainting can signal a serious health condition. Medical evaluation is recommended after a fainting spell.

Grief

Grief is a part of our lives. Children may grieve the loss of a friend because of a move, their parents' divorce, or a death in the family. In some cases, this experience can affect a child's life forever. Homeopathy can prevent that. As in all other cases, there are many homeopathic remedies that help with grief. I've treated a number of children in this state and find that the single most frequently required remedy is *Ignatia amara*.

Of course, *Ignatia* isn't going to be the only remedy you'll ever need for this problem, but in my opinion, it's the one you'll most frequently find helpful. If the picture that the child develops doesn't fit this remedy, simply don't give it.

- *Ignatia amara*. The key to understanding the state that requires this remedy is hysteria. The child tries to hold back crying, which results in sobbing and eventually in hysterical loud crying. Also, the child doesn't want to be consoled. Typically, children feel a lump in the throat and sigh frequently. They become easily offended and very defensive and touchy. They may also become rude, critical, and suspicious. In addition, they may develop other hysterical symptoms, like numbness, headache, back spasms, or even paralysis. Any ailment that develops after grief sets in may respond extremely well to this remedy.

I've given *Ignatia* 200C to teenagers and young adults as a constitutional remedy and in a few cases have received reports that they had a breakup shortly after that and reacted in a calm, composed way. I recommend giving one dose of this remedy about fifteen minutes before giving someone bad news (such as, "Your father and I are getting divorced" or "Your grandfather just passed away"). You can repeat the dose once or twice, if there's only a partial effect, or if the initial improvement begins to disappear. I would call *Ignatia* "*Arnica* for a broken heart."

Just remember, if a person becomes quiet and appears frozen after grief or develops other symptoms that don't fit the *Ignatia* profile, contact a homeopath or a mental health professional.

There are also rare cases of children becoming very depressed and even suicidal after significant losses. Seek professional help immediately, and do not leave such a child without supervision until help is obtained.

Food Poisoning

The following remedies may be useful when dealing with food poisoning:

- *Arsenicum album.* Always think of this remedy first in cases of food poisoning. Signs include diarrhea accompanied by anxiety. If the child vomits, he becomes fearful; the child often struggles not to vomit because of this fear. The vomit may be bitter. The child is restless, very weak, and thirsty for small sips of cold drinks. Frequently, you'll hear complaints about burning pains—don't overestimate the importance of this symptom. Many children have difficulties distinguishing the exact characteristics and location of their pain.
- *Urtica urens.* *Urtica* is an excellent remedy for shellfish poisoning, especially if it's accompanied by severe itching and hives.
- *Veratrum album.* *Veratrum* is good for the kind of severe vomiting that's frequently described as *projectile vomiting*, when it's accompanied by diarrhea. So what you have is simultaneous vomiting and diarrhea. Other indicators are extreme prostration (the person cannot even wiggle a finger) and cold sweat, especially on the forehead.

Natural Disasters and Terror

Unfortunately, terrorism has become a regular part of daily life in recent years. I witnessed the events of 9-11 in New York and treated a number of victims for acute and chronic post-traumatic stress disorder (PTSD). I've worked with kids from crime-ridden, inner-city neighborhoods who have seen their family and friends shot right in front of them. Now, as I'm writing this book, the world is also dealing with the results of a disastrous tsunami in South Asia. People in the directly affected countries are suffering from PTSD. Homeopathy literally performs miracles for these survivors. It also helps tremendously to overcome grief in cases of loss. (See the corresponding previous section.)

Certainly, an experienced homeopath will be able to provide effective assistance. But finding a trained homeopath quickly in a disastrous situation can be difficult. You may need to self-treat until help can be reached. Here are a few very frequently indicated remedies. The symptoms you'll need to consider to make an appropriate selection are usually so severe and so clear that finding the correct remedy is easy.

- *Aconitum napellus*. If I had to name only one remedy for victims of terror and natural disasters, this remedy would be my first choice. The most characteristic symptoms of an *Aconitum* state are severe fear, frequently accompanied by an unexplainable, vivid sense or even a conviction of imminent death; restlessness; and agitation. The victim looks scared and has very small pupils.

This remedy is often indicated during the first hours after an event. But I've actually seen a number of cases in which a person remained in this state for years and then was cured by *Aconitum*.

- *Arsenicum album*. The key to understanding this remedy is anxiety. Victims are very anxious, restless, and fidgety. They constantly call for help and need to be reassured; they need company. They may become chilly and feel much worse after midnight. They're unable to sleep. They may develop diarrhea from severe anxiety. They're also thirsty for small amounts of cold drinks.

• *Stramonium*. Indications of this state include terrible nightmares (for example, when a child wakes up scared and remembers the dream) and night terrors (for example, when a child wakes up morbidly scared but doesn't remember the dream). Children also may develop violent behavior after a significant terrorizing experience. This violence seems to come in outbursts, without any apparent premeditation. They also become afraid of the dark, dogs and other animals, and water. Some children begin to stammer, and some may exhibit various grimaces and twitches.

In addition to homeopathy, providing debriefing and psychological treatment for the victims and their families after a calamitous event is very important.

Sunstroke and Heat Prostration

Children are susceptible to sunstroke and heat prostration because of their small body mass. Sunstroke presents itself very acutely with a full, extremely rapid pulse. Heat prostration develops more gradually, and the presentation is less dramatic than in sunstroke, but it's equally dangerous. When either condition occurs, the victim must be put in the shade and cooled off as quickly as possible. Remember this: if the skin is dry and very hot, or if the body temperature is rising very quickly, the situation may be life threatening. First aid is to pour cool water on the victim, apply ice, and give the child ice-cold drinks. Calling 9-1-1 is a must.

While waiting for help to arrive, give a remedy.

• *Belladonna*. Indications include high fever, burning dry and flushed skin, enlarged pupils, and a very strong and rapid pulse.
• *Cuprum metallicum* (copper). Indications include the same symptoms as for *Veratrum album*, plus cramps.
• *Glonoine* (nitroglycerine). Indications include the same symptoms as for *Belladonna*, but with the addition of a terrible, bursting headache.

- *Veratrum album.* This remedy is most useful in cases of heat exhaustion, which usually result from dehydration. The pulse is not as pounding as in sunstroke (it doesn't go higher than a hundred beats per minute), and the skin is cold and clammy. The victim is pale, weak, and nauseous.

Surgery

Frequently, surgical procedures are planned. More often, surgery is the treatment of choice for an emergency. Of course, most parents would perceive their child's surgery as an emergency situation even if it were planned.

- *Aconitum napellus.* This remedy is helpful for shock and fright before and after surgery, if a child is morbidly scared and— especially— convinced that he or she will die during the operation. I've known quite a few adults who felt this way, too. One dose of 30C can make a huge difference. (Compare with *Gelsemium.*)
- *Arnica montana.* The stress of surgery is so profound that an overwhelming majority of humans go into the state that responds well to this particular remedy before and after surgery. This is true for general trauma, too. Arnica is especially good for surgery that involves trauma to a combination of skin, muscles, and bones, like orthopedic and plastic surgery. Certainly, it works for complicated dental surgery and many other types of surgery. My patients swear by it.

Please remember that giving a remedy too much and too frequently may cause a proving. In the case of *Arnica*, it could mean more bruising and bleeding than otherwise. Here's what I recommend to parents: give your child *Arnica* 200C the morning of surgery, another dose on waking up from anesthesia (or right after surgery is finished), and one more dose at night. This schedule certainly can be interrupted if the child feels fine.

Alpine Pharmaceuticals produces an interesting product called *SinEcch,* which contains several doses of *Arnica* at different strengths, packaged to be consumed in a particular order. Simple instructions are provided. The remedy is placed in capsules that can be swallowed like a conventional medication. This preparation is becoming popular among plastic surgeons and is appropriate for anyone undergoing serious surgical procedures that require *Arnica*. It's especially good for nihilistic teenagers, who don't want to take "weird pills."

• *Gelsemium sempervirens*. This works well for severe anxiety before surgery. The child could be trembling with fear and feel weak. (Compare with the *Aconitum* state, where the reaction is very strong and includes terror and a strong fear of death.)

• *Phosphorus*. This remedy helps relieve bad effects of anesthesia, like disorientation, anxiety, nausea, and vomiting. It's helpful for nausea and vomiting after abdominal surgery.

Common Problems Easily Treated with Homeopathy

Homeopathy is extremely effective in treating common childhood infections, some of which all children experience at one time or another. This section discusses the childhood infections chicken pox, measles, rubella, mumps, parvovirous, and mononucleosis.

These illnesses are becoming more and more uncommon due to vaccinations. Although it's a rare occurrence, they may cause significant distress in your child. The beginning of these illnesses looks like a common cold or a flu and should be treated with remedies described in the next section ("Colds and Flu"). When the correctly chosen remedies work right away, you might not even know that your child had chicken pox or measles. The specific remedies listed here are also very helpful. You should always get in touch with your physician right away. All of these diseases are viral, and antibiotics don't help in the initial stages of the illness. However, the homeopathic remedies listed here provide effective relief for specific symptoms of each childhood disease. As with any other illness, you should not try many various remedies. Allow a homeopath to deal with the situation if your initial efforts fail. If, despite your best efforts, bacterial infection complicates the situation, allow your pediatrician or a family physician to use his or her skills to improve your child's condition.

There are a few remedies that are considered to be specific for particular complaints associated with these diseases. I will list the ones that I have found helpful in my practice, including specific characteristics for the remedies used in the treatment of colds and fever.

Chicken Pox

The discomfort is caused by eruptions that look like little pimples (blisters) and appear on the trunk first, than face and head in crops. The illness lasts for about ten days, but the incubation period (time between the exposure and the appearance of first symptoms) is the longest of all childhood infections: two to three weeks. This disease is highly contagious, from a few days before the appearance of eruptions until the last blister scabs over. It is caused by the varicella virus, which belongs to the herpes family of viruses. These viruses can remain in the body for many years and become reactivated with stress in adults causing shingles (herpes zoster). The majority of cases are mild, but some children may develop severe symptoms and have complications.

- *Antimonium crudum.* This remedy is almost a specific for chicken pox. The child is very irritable and does not want to be touched in any way, including bathing, or even looked at. The tongue is usually coated white. The child who needs this remedy is almost identical to the child who needs *Chamomilla*. It is very specific for chicken pox; *Chamomilla* is not.
- *Antimonium tartaricum.* The child is also irritable and whining and has wet rattling cough when the phlegm in the chest is difficult to expel. The child wants company. The eruptions are large pustules.
- *Pulsatilla nigricans.* The child is sweet and weepy, wants to be comforted. What a difference from the *Antimonium* family!
- *Rhus toxicondenron.* This remedy is useful when there are extreme itching and extreme mental and physical restlessness. The

child is frequently thirsty for milk. (Do not concentrate on this symptom; it is only confirmatory to the rest of the picture.)

- *Sulphur.* The itching is pretty bad. The child is very thirsty for cold drinks and is hungry, taking more that he can eat.

Measles (Seven-Day Measles)

You probably know this illness by its typical skin rash. But in actuality, measles is mainly a respiratory infection. Infants are generally protected from measles for six to eight months after birth due to immunities that were passed on from their mothers. Older children are usually immunized with the mumps, measles, and rubella (MMR) vaccine. The first manifestations of measles are a very high fever (up to 105 degrees Fahrenheit); a runny nose; red, very-sensitive-to-light eyes; and a dry, hacking cough. Interestingly, the fever peaks with the appearance of the rash. The rash begins on the forehead and spreads downward over the face, neck, and body. Usually, it takes three days to make its way down to the feet. Symptoms subside once the rash reaches the feet. The rash fades in the same order that it appeared, from forehead to feet. Isn't it a neat illustration of Hering's Law?

Flat blotches that often merge with one another, especially on the face and shoulders, represent the measles rash. It stays, from beginning to end, for about seven days. One special identifying sign of measles is Koplik's spots. These are small, irregularly shaped spots with blue-white centers that are found inside the mouth. Koplik's spots may be noticed one to two days before the measles rash appears on the skin.

The majority of children recover from this illness completely. But measles can lead to many different complications: croup, bronchitis, ear infections, pneumonia, conjunctivitis, myocarditis (inflammation of the heart muscle), hepatitis, and encephalitis (inflammation of the brain). The latter condition manifests in the form of seizures, confusion, and unconsciousness.

Please remember, if you suspect measles in your child, contact the physician right away. You still can give a homeopathic remedy and get excellent results. Better safe than sorry. Measles is most contagious two to four days before the appearance of the rash.

- *Aconitum napellus*. *Aconitum* is useful in the very beginning of the illness. The child is scared and restless. There's aching pain in the eyes, which are sensitive to light. The child also has a profuse stream of tears and nasal discharge and a croupy cough.
- *Belladonna*. The child is bothered by light, noises, and jarring. He may be confused. He has a flushed face, sore throat, and no thirst.
- *Bryonia alba*. Not wanting to move is the typical characteristic of this child. The slightest motion provokes dry cough. The child is thirsty for large amounts of cold water. Interestingly, this remedy speeds up the appearance of the rash, thus relieving the symptoms. Use it only if symptoms point toward this remedy. Do not give it just because you want the rash to come out. As with all other homeopathic remedies, *Bryonia* will work only if it's properly indicated.
- *Dulcamara*. Use this remedy for cough and all other characteristic symptoms of measles that appear following rainy, wet, cold weather.
- *Euphrasia officinalis*. Symptoms include conjunctivitis with profuse irritating tears that leave marks on the face, pus in the eyes, and a croupy cough during the day. It's made better from lying down.
- *Ferrum phosphoricum*. Use this for measles with a very high fever, general malaise, and no specific symptoms. Do not underestimate the power of this remedy in early stages of the illness.
- *Gelsemium sempervirens*. The child in this state has severe weakness. Her eyelids are heavy and she can even be lethargic. There's no thirst. The cough is croupy and hoarse.
- *Pulsatilla nigricans*. *Pulsatilla* is useful in the later stages of measles. This remedy is considered a specific for the aftereffects of measles if the typical symptoms are present: child is weepy and wants attention and consolation. Cough is dry at night and loose during the day. The child may complain of earache. The eyes are watery and can be inflamed with pus, which makes the eyelids stick. All symptoms are worse at dusk.

Rubella (German Measles or Three-Day Measles)

Rubella is usually a mild disease that is caused by the rubella virus, which is distinct from the virus that causes measles. It primarily affects the skin and lymph nodes in the back of the neck and behind the ears. In children, it's usually transmitted by secretions from the nose or throat. It can also pass through a pregnant woman's bloodstream to her unborn child. Although not a dangerous disease in children, rubella infection in a pregnant woman presents significant dangers to the fetus, as the virus easily crosses the placenta and is known to cause severe congenital problems in developing babies.

Children infected with rubella before birth are at risk for growth retardation; mental retardation; malformations of the heart and eyes; deafness; and liver, spleen, and bone marrow problems. If you are planning on getting pregnant, make sure your doctor checks your rubella *titer* (concentration of antibodies). This simple blood test will show whether you are immune to this illness or not. If pregnant, homeopathic treatment may not resolve the complications of the fetus. No research on this issue is available. Some homeopaths suggest using a rubella nosode for prophylaxis of this illness, but there's no data behind the idea.

In young children, rubella infections usually begin with a low-grade fever (99 to 100 degrees Fahrenheit) and swollen, tender lymph nodes, which are usually located in the back of the neck or behind the ears. A rash appears on the second or the third day. It begins on the face and spreads downward. As it spreads down the body, it usually clears on the face (another example of Hering's Law in action). Parents usually realize that the child is sick after they see the first signs of this rash.

The rubella rash looks like many other viral rashes. It can be presented by either pink or light red spots, which may merge and form evenly colored patches. The rash can itch and lasts up to three days.

Homeopathic treatment of this illness is very similar to treatment for common colds. Don't forget about *Ferrum phosphoricum* if you can't find any specific symptoms.

Mumps

The chances of your child contracting the mumps are very low. Before the vaccine, which was created in 1967, up to two hundred thousand cases a year occurred in the United States. Now there are fewer than three hundred cases a year. Mumps mostly affects children ages five to fourteen, but the proportion of young adults who become infected has been slowly rising over the last two decades. Mumps is uncommon in children younger than one year. One attack of mumps almost always gives lifelong protection.

The virus that causes this infection mainly affects the parotid salivary glands, which produce saliva for the mouth. They are located toward the back of each cheek, in the area between the ear and jaw. In cases of mumps, these glands typically swell and become painful. As a result, the child looks like a cute little guinea pig or a hamster with food in its cheeks. Medical historians argue over whether the name *mumps* comes from an old word for *lump* or an old word for *mumble*.

Be aware that other infections can also cause swelling in the salivary glands and might make you think that a child has had mumps more than once.

Mumps is usually pretty mild in its course, and it is benign. In rare cases, mumps may result in encephalitis (inflammation of the brain) and meningitis (inflammation of the lining of the brain and spinal cord). Symptoms appear in the first week after the parotid glands begin to swell. They may include high fever, stiff neck, headache, nausea, vomiting, drowsiness, convulsions, and other signs of brain involvement. In cases like that, call 9-1-1 or go to the nearest ER.

Mumps in adolescent boys may result in the development of orchitis, an inflammation of the testicles. Usually, one testicle becomes swollen and painful about seven to ten days after the parotids swell. This is accompanied by a high fever, shaking chills, headache, nausea, vomiting, and abdominal pain, which can sometimes be mistaken for appendicitis, if the right testicle is affected. In some cases, both testicles are involved. Testicular pain and swelling tend to go away around the time the fever passes. Some parents are concerned about the possibility of a boy becoming sterile. According to the literature, sterility is a rare complication even if both testicles are involved.

- *Apis mellifica.* The swelling is soft and tender. There is no thirst. Some children may become irritable and even angry.
- *Belladonna.* The child may be restless and confused. The face is red and flushed, and the eyes are sensitive to light. Although high fever may be present, the child isn't thirsty.
- *Bryonia alba.* The child may be irritable and wants to be left alone. The swelling is hard (compare with *Apis*) and feels tender. The child doesn't want to move, as the slightest motion of the head causes pain. The lips are dry and cracked. The child is also thirsty for large amounts of cold water.
- *Mercurius solubilis.* The child has profuse salivation with foul, offensive breath and may have bleeding gums. The testes may be also inflamed. There's profuse perspiration. The child may become suspicious.
- *Pulsatilla nigricans.* This remedy is very helpful if the disease lingers. It may spread to testes. The child presents with a typical picture of the remedy: weepy, whining, no thirst, and craving open air. Symptoms may be changeable.

Mononucleosis

Mononucleosis, or mono, has a nickname: the "kissing disease." It's an illness generally caused by the Epstein-Barr virus (EBV), which is transmitted through saliva, and is occasionally caused by cytomegalovirus, a close relative of EBV. Young children can be infected from the saliva of playmates or family members. Adolescents typically spread the virus through kissing (hence its once popular nickname). When people think of infectious mono, extreme tiredness is one of the major symptoms they associate with it. Although clinical markers of the disease are swollen lymph nodes in the neck and armpits and an enlarged spleen, they are frequently absent at the onset. Mono begins with fever, sore throat, and sore muscles.

Children and adolescents diagnosed with sore throats are usually given antibiotics such as ampicillin or amoxicillin, especially if their tonsils are swollen, even though these are not helpful for the viruses that cause mono. Frequently, these drugs cause a pink rash to develop all over the body.

Most children recover from mono completely, but some have complications, such as blood disorders leading to lowered numbers of red and white blood cells because of decreased production of these cells by the bone marrow or destruction of red blood cells (hemolytic anemia). They may also develop Bell's palsy, a usually temporary condition caused by the inflammation of a facial nerve, which leads to weakness or paralysis of the facial muscles on one side of the face. There is another, also rare, complication called Guillain-Barré syndrome, which can paralyze muscles. Other rare complications include rupture of the spleen, inflammation of the heart muscle (myocarditis), and involvement of the central nervous system (aseptic meningitis and encephalitis).

Infection with the virus usually provides long-lasting immunity. Studies show that most people have been infected with EBV at some point in their lives, and most have few or no symptoms of viral infection. A vaccine for EBV hasn't been developed yet.

One of the most unfortunate frequent complications of mono is long-term weakness, which is especially characteristic for adolescents. I've seen a number of cases of youths with this problem, and I've learned that homeopathy can be helpful in overcoming it.

You may be able to stop mononucleosis from developing by using one of the remedies for treatment of colds, flu, and fever at an early stage in the illness. (See the next section, "Colds and Flu.") One of them may also be very useful in helping your child recover from mono. If mono develops, consult a homeopath.

A physician should also be involved from the beginning of the illness to make a correct diagnosis—supported by blood work—and to prevent severe complications.

Colds and Flu

This is probably the single area of medicine where laypersons feel that they are most able to treat themselves and their families. In most supermarkets, the OTC section for colds and flu is several shelves long. Many varieties of medications for fevers, coughs, and congestion are displayed and seem as though they're being purchased by the pound. Unfortunately, even the best of these popular concoctions are suppressive at their best, and all of them have numerous side effects, especially in children.

The best achievements by conventional medicine in the area of prevention are flu vaccines, which have all the disadvantages and limitations of any other vaccination.

There are also numerous herbal preparations, some of which can be efficacious in addressing minor colds. The trouble is that they have to be taken continually for the duration of the cold and flu season and also may pose certain risks. Overmedication with any substance is not a good idea, even if it's a natural substance.

It's a bad idea to send sick children to school. For some reason, many parents feel that a simple cold with a low-grade or no fever doesn't justify allowing a child to stay at home. In reality, sending a sick child to school does a lot of damage. First of all, the child doesn't get time to rest and recover from the illness. Second, that sick child brings myriad viruses to school and infects other children. Third, during the cold and flu season other students are coming to school sick and exposing that child to illnesses. This creates a free market of different types and subtypes of viruses being easily exchanged between different vulnerable children.

Of course, many working parents are compelled to send their sick children to school because they don't have a caring relative, such as a grandmother or another adult helper, to take care of the children. But if you have an option, you should utilize it.

Simple Solutions for Colds and Flu

There are two hugely popular homeopathic products for flu on the market: *Oscillococcinum* and *Influenzinum*. Both are used in an allopathic manner: the same remedy for everyone. There is no individualization of treatment. Still, many people find them effective. Of course, if your child is undergoing homeopathic treatment, you shouldn't use these remedies, or better yet, you should ask the treating homeopath for an opinion. If your child isn't under a homeopath's care, and you've had the time and energy to read this book, you could try an individual approach instead of these products.

Some people (or should I say the majority of people?) like simple solutions. Here is the information on these two "simple" solutions:

• *Oscillococcinum* (also called *Anas barbariae hepatis et cordis extractum* 200C). *Oscillococcinum* is an anomaly in the homeopathic *Materia Medica* because it is one of the relatively few proprietary single-remedy preparations. The French company Boiron licenses the name. Whereas most remedies in France are made using Hahnemannian dilutions, production of *Oscillococcinum* is done by the Korsakoff method. Interestingly, it is the only homeopathic medicine authorized for routine distribution in France in a dilution above 30C.

The reason for this exception is that *Oscillococcinum* is the number one OTC flu medication in France. It's also been popular in other European countries and presently is growing in popularity in the United States.

The history of the discovery of this remedy is quite interesting. A French physician, Joseph Roy, M.D., introduced it in the 1930s. He thought he'd discovered oscillating bacteria in the blood of patients who had the flu and many other illnesses, including cancer. He called this phenomenon oscillococcus (meaning "oscillating round bacteria" in Latin). To date, we don't know what Roy saw under his microscope. Certainly, it wasn't a flu virus (you cannot see viruses under a regular optical microscope), nor was it any bacteria we know.

For his homeopathic preparation, Roy decided to use a particular type of duck that's used in France to prepare delicious duck breast. That's why the remedy is designated with the Latin name *Anas barbariae hepatis et cordis extractum*, meaning an autolysate of Barbary duck liver and heart. Interestingly, it has been shown that fowl is a major reservoir of human influenza viruses. Certainly, this remedy is not the first example, and not the last example, of a medication being introduced on the basis of a wrong theory—and then proven to be effective.

The British Journal of Clinical Pharmacology published a large-scale double-blind, placebo-controlled trial in which 487 patients were recruited by 149 general practitioners (mostly nonhomeopaths) in the Rhone-Alpes region of France during the January to February 1987 influenza epidemic. According to this report, 17 percent of the active treatment group fully recovered, compared with 10 percent of the placebo group. This difference is statistically significant ($p = 0.03$, X2 test).

Further analysis showed that the effect of *Oscillococcinum* peaked at thirty-six hours, when 40 percent of recoveries were attributable to the treatment. It was most effective in younger patients (68 percent of recoveries within forty-eight hours in the under-thirties were due to treatment) and when the illness was relatively mild (52 percent of the recoveries from illnesses classified as mild or moderate were due to treatment). Patients on active treatment used significantly less other treatment for pain and fever (50 versus 41 percent). They also judged the active treatment more efficacious than placebo (61 versus 49 percent).

According to the package directions, *Oscillococcinum* should be used at the first sign of a cold or flu. Instructions are easy to follow and printed on the package. Some people swear by it; others don't find it effective. But it's certainly better than even less-specific OTC drugs. It might be a good choice of a remedy for a rebellious teenager who doesn't believe in anything and doesn't even want to spend a minute talking to you. Obviously, a rebel would prefer *Oscillococcinum* to anything allopathic. According to the study just described, it may prevent the development of a full-blown cold or flu. Of course, it can also be helpful in keeping adults healthy.

• *Influenzinum* is a preparation of a current flu vaccine in the 9C potency. Like *Oscillococcinum*, it's popular in Europe for flu prevention. It's being marketed as an alternative to the flu shot for ages two and up. But there isn't much scientific evidence of its efficacy. According to a ten-year study done in collaboration with twenty-three French homeopathic doctors, it has been effective in 90 percent of cases. I am not familiar with the design of the research study. All I can say is that these numbers seem to be too optimistic. Together with *Oscillococcinum*, this is yet another example of the allopathic use of a homeopathically prepared substance. Nonetheless I must admit that I've met people (usually from France) who swear by it.

Various homeopathic companies sell *Influenzinum* under different brand names as well as its generic name. The instructions are the same for all of these products. It is recommended to dissolve one dose (the entire contents of a tube) under the tongue each week for four weeks and then to wait for another three weeks before dissolving the contents of one final tube under the tongue.

Like *Oscillococcinum*, the routine use of this remedy, especially in children who are already under homeopathic care, isn't a good idea.

Homeopathy for Colds and Flu

You'll notice that the majority of the remedies described in this section are exactly the same as in the section called "Fever." The reason is simple. Very often, fever is the first response a healthy child has to a cold or flu. By the time you get to see a doctor, the acute characteristic state that arises at the very beginning of an illness is over; the opportunity to halt the development of a bad cold or flu has been missed.

You may be at the forefront of a chain of responses, so to speak, and if you clearly see the signs of a remedy and give it to your child right away, a lot of trouble can be saved. We are reminded of how much trouble there can be each time we don't get the remedy right and our children go on to develop coughs and sinus problems. To make things easier on you, I've decided not to send you back to the "Fever" section but to present all the remedies here, so you can easily choose the one your child needs.

- *Aconitum napellus.* Use this if the onset is very sudden, as frequently happens after a child is exposed to cold wind. Often significant chills precede this fever, and it usually rises in the evening or at night. The child is very thirsty and the pupils are small. (Compare with *Belladonna.*)

The mental symptoms are excitement with fear and restlessness. If the child isn't excited and restless, *Aconitum* probably isn't a good choice. The physical symptoms are a thirst for cold and having one cheek red, another pale (similar to *Chamomilla*).

- *Arsenicum album.* In this state, the child is restless, but unlike the *Aconitum* state, it isn't from terror; it's from significant anxiety. This remedy is frequently indicated for colds and flu with diarrhea and vomiting. The child complains of burning pains (for example, in the throat), which are made better by warm applications. Burning better from warmth is a symptom that's unique to this remedy. The child is also thirsty for cold water, but only in small sips. (Compare with *Aconitum, Bryonia,* and *Phosphorus* states, in which the child has a thirst for large amounts of cold water.) The face is hot; the rest of the body is cold. Head symptoms are better from cold, symptoms in the rest of the body from heat.

- *Belladonna.* The picture is usually very clear. Use for a cold or a flu with a very rapid onset and very high fever (up to 105 degrees). The child may be confused. It does not always happen, but the child often looks somewhat "off." Eyes are glassy. Pupils are large. (Compare with *Aconitum.*) In some cases, you may notice slight twitching of the face and the body or even febrile seizures.

The face and body are hot to the touch, and the hands and feet are cold. (Don't get stuck on this last symptom. If it's there, go for it. If not, look at everything else). The child has no thirst or specifically asks for lemonade or lemons. Sometimes the child initially has chills. These usually occur in the afternoon and begin in the arms or in the abdomen.

• *Bryonia alba*. Fever usually develops slowly. Interestingly, the chills (if they happen) begin either at 9 A.M. or 9 P.M. and start in the fingertips, toes, or lips. Children in this state complain of pains and want to be absolutely still, quiet, left alone. They may become confused, then they are characteristically scared that they aren't at home and ask to go home. They have an incredible thirst for large amounts of very cold water. At times, their thirst in unquenchable. When chilly, the face is white. When the fever rises, the face becomes deep red. As cough sets in, it becomes very painful. Even a slight motion can set it off. A headache is usually in the left side in the front, or it is all the way in the back of the head.

• *Eupatorium perfoliatum*. The main feature of this state is severe pains and aching of muscles and bones. This state could look similar to *Bryonia*, but actually it's quite different, as it doesn't have a feature of getting irritated by the slightest motion. The *Eupatorium* child might not want to move due to pains and aches, although it's possible. A *Bryonia* child wouldn't even entertain a thought of moving. The fever is high and the child is thirsty for cold liquids.

• *Ferrum phosphoricum*. Use this remedy for a high fever that lasts for days, when there's a gradual onset of the illness. Usually, there are no local symptoms, but at times the child may have a headache or a sore throat all on the right side.

• *Gelsemium sempervirens*. Use for fever accompanied by tremendous weakness and sleepiness. The child can be trembling from weakness and sometimes cannot even open the eyes. Chills are running up and down the child's back, and the back of the head feels very heavy. Often there's an occipital headache. The child has blurry vision and at times even double vision. The limbs are also heavy. The child is not thirsty.

- *Nux vomica.* Use this when the child is extremely sensitive to cold, light, noises, and odors and is also very irritable. In this state, a high fever sets in quickly, but the child wants to be covered and asks for warm drinks and food. The child absolutely cannot tolerate anything cold. (Compare with *Bryonia.*) In addition, the child may become sleepless. One of the characteristic features of this remedy is that people who need it, no matter what their complaints, feel better from warmth and rest.

- *Phosphorus.* You should think about this remedy if a child with a high fever (103 to 104 degrees) remains active and appears perfectly well. The child is also thirsty for cold drinks, is chilly, has night sweats, and has a cold moving into the chest.

- *Rhus toxicodendron.* The child who needs this remedy has aching throughout the body, which is made better from constant motion. Often this child is anxious and restless. There can be stiffness with improvement from stretching. The child is thirsty for small sips of water. A very characteristic symptom is a red triangle on the very tip of the tongue. The child may also have a cold sore during fever.

Other Conditions Where Homeopathy Can Help

This section discusses a variety of conditions where homeopathy can help your child.

Colic

This term refers to infants with digestive upset, when the baby is crying, doubled up, and passing gas. Usually, this is a self-limiting condition. A lot of babies have it and outgrow it by the age of four months. But it is painful to the infant, and watching your baby suffering can be very distressing. Please make sure to consult with a physician if this problem doesn't go away very quickly, or returns after only a few hours of relief. The following remedies might help your baby:

- *Belladonna*. In this state, the baby has a distended, hot abdomen. At times, you might see protruding intestines. The infant is hypersensitive to noise and the least jarring motion. The child can be angry and strike at you. Symptoms are made better by bending backward and also by lying on the abdomen. (Compare with the *Colocynthis* state, in which the baby is angry but made better from bending forward.)
- *Bryonia alba*. The baby absolutely doesn't want to be moved or touched! Even if you want to carry your baby or give your baby a warm bottle, he will scream and fight with you. The emotional picture can be similar to *Chamomilla* (screaming and fighting), but you'll clearly see that a child who needs *Chamomilla* wants to be carried all the time. That's different from the primary issue in the *Bryonia* child.
- *Chamomilla*. The baby who needs this remedy has lots of gas and green diarrhea that smells like spoiled eggs. The child is hot, thirsty, very demanding, and *capricious* (for example, he refuses what he initially asked for). The baby is much better if carried around continuously and will start screaming again if put down. It is a remedy frequently indicated for infants.
- *Colocynthis*. Children who benefit from this remedy get better from hard pressure and bending double, often demonstrated by relief when laid over the seated parent's leg. Their pains can be provoked or get worse from anger. The child is usually restless with pain.

Please note that children who get better from bending backward benefit from *Belladonna* or from *Dioscorea villosa* (wild yam), which isn't in the kit you've built because it is indicated so infrequently. Also always make a point to compare this remedy with *Magnesia phosphorica*.

- *Magnesia phosphorica*. This remedy relieves colic pains that are much better from warm applications and bending double. Unlike *Colocynthis*, hard pressure is not as helpful as warm applications.

Cough

Many self-help books on homeopathy offer instructions on how to treat coughs. In reality, treating a cough can be difficult for a layperson.

As a parent, please ensure that a physician sees your child with a persistent cough. You really don't want to overlook a serious condition like bronchitis or pneumonia. Although homeopathy can cure these illnesses, you really have to know what you're doing when you attempt it. However, if your physician tells you, after the examination, that there's nothing serious wrong with your child and then begins giving you advice on OTC cough medications, it's a golden opportunity for you to come in and try homeopathy.

As always, give your child the best remedy you can pick while you are waiting to see the doctor. Sometimes it takes a few hours to get in for an appointment. If you win, the prize is going to be huge: no cough and no other symptoms of a cold.

Actually, if you catch the very beginning of the cold with a correct remedy, a cough may be stopped in its tracks. But sometimes, you won't see your child until after school when the initials stages of a cold have passed already. If an initial dose of the remedy you've chosen doesn't bring any relief, consult your homeopath.

I've seen many cases when a child (or an adult) had typical symptoms indicating a particular remedy but came to me laden with heavy-duty medications on board already (antibiotics or hormones). Homeopathy still can be very helpful at these times, and it promptly eliminates a cough. As I was writing this book, for example, I saw a patient who actually has been with me for over a year. Sam originally came for depression. It went away after homeopathic treatment, and he would come every now and then with minor problems. Although homeopathy always worked for him, Sam remained "a strong believer in conventional medicine," as he put it.

Around Christmas time, he had a pretty severe cold. But he felt uneasy about giving me a call. He decided "to tough it out" and didn't take any medicine at all until the New Year. On January second, he developed a severe cough that was unbearable. It was dry and would get much worse each time he went out in the cold or tried to talk. It was also worse at night and when he lay down, and it was especially awful if Sam attempted to sleep in his favorite position on his left side.

Another peculiar symptom was an almost constant tickling behind his sternum and in his throat. Sam went to his family physician, who prescribed a powerful antibiotic. After ten days of treatment nothing happened. A chest X ray showed no pneumonia. A covering physician, who this patient saw after the course of the antibiotics was finished, then prescribed prednisone tablets for five days along with a cough-suppressing medicine. After two days on this treatment, Sam's cough was still there. It did not change a bit.

At this point, Sam realized that something was wrong with his treatment and made an emergency appointment with me. About ten minutes into the interview, I clearly saw a picture of *Rumex*, one of the remedies that is described later in the chapter.

Now, I didn't want Sam to stop taking the prednisone (a hormone) abruptly. Once you have a significant dose, it has to be tapered off slowly, and Sam had the right instructions from his physician. So I advised Sam to take *Rumex* 30C twice a day for the next four days, which was the duration of his prednisone protocol, and to stop taking the remedy earlier if his cough got 100 percent better. In cases when antibiotics or hormones are prescribed, a remedy has to be taken more frequently because the allopathic drug constantly antidotes—or reverses—the action of the remedy. I also advised Sam to stop taking the cough suppressant.

Sam called me the next day. After only one dose of *Rumex* 30C, he had been able to sleep through the night on his left side! After two more doses, the whole episode of coughing was over.

Please don't get discouraged if you need to give your children some conventional drugs when they're sick. Even then, homeopathy may still help speed up their healing process. Sam's situation is a very common one in our society.

A cough can be either dry (no discharge) or productive (with mucus). Remedies for these two types of cough will be presented separately.

Dry Cough (No Discharge). Very commonly needed remedies for dry cough are the following:

- *Bryonia alba.* Use *Bryonia* for very painful, dry coughing that arises with each ever-so-slight movement, or even with every breath. The child who needs this remedy may be afraid to take a breath. The child often holds the chest and the head each time he coughs to prevent pain. Symptoms are made worse by bending the head backward (compare with *Hepar sulphur* and *Spongia*), eating, and swallowing. Symptoms are made better in the open air.
- *Rumex crispus.* This is the main remedy for tickling, irritating coughs that feel worse from cold air (compare with *Coccus cacti*) and worse from entering or leaving a warm room (that is, out to cold, or in from cold). But the cough is better if the child stays in a warm room for a while. Symptoms also feel worse from undressing. Symptoms are made better from turning to the right side (similar to *Phosphorus*). To confirm this remedy, press very lightly in the pit of the throat. The child who needs *Rumex* will have a paroxysm of coughing.
- *Spongia tosta. Spongia* is for a cough that is better from eating or drinking, warm food or drinks, and from bending the head forward. (Compare with *Hepar sulphur.*)

There are a number of remedies that share the same symptom as their important, key feature: *they're made worse by lying down.* Let's see what makes them different.

- *Causticum.* This state has an irritating cough with tickling in the throat. The child feels like there is mucus in the chest. She tries to cough deeper to raise the mucus, but there is no expectoration. Often the child must swallow the mucus. The child is frequently hoarse and especially tries to clear her throat in the morning. The cough is worse from bending the head forward (compare with *Spongia*), and from cold drinks. Interestingly, it's also better in rainy weather. This cough completely clears up during the day. There may be involuntary urination during the cough.

• *Coccus cacti.* Use this remedy for cough that occurs in hard, short paroxysms. This cough may end with a lot of mucus, or often no mucus. It is made worse from heat, being in warm rooms, and consuming warm drinks and food. Symptoms are better from cold open air, and from cold drinks and food. (Compare with *Phosphorus* and *Rumex.*)

• *Drosera rotundifolia.* Use this for paroxysms of violent, hard, dry coughing. This is a suffocative, very painful cough, which becomes worse the moment the child's head touches the pillow at night. But it may be better from lying down during the day. Symptoms worsen from eating or drinking. (Compare with *Spongia.*)

There is one remedy that helps when there is a very *significant improvement on lying down.*

• *Euphrasia officinalis.* This remedy is most frequently indicated for allergic coughs. Use when the child coughs all day but has absolutely no cough at night. It feels much better on lying down and eating. It feels worse from talking.

Moist Cough (Productive). The following remedies are effective in treating a moist cough.

• *Antimonium tartaricum. Antimonium* is frequently indicated for toddlers and even younger children with rattling coughs, when you get an impression that the chest of the child is filled with mucus and yet no mucus comes out. The child is frequently irritable and doesn't want to be touched. Symptoms are worse from eating and lying still. They're also worse at night, especially after 10 P.M.

• *Hepar sulphur.* This cough is dry at night, but loose in the morning. (Compare with *Pulsatilla.*) The mucus is thick and yellow. Symptoms are made worse by anything cold: air, drinks, food, and so on. The child starts coughing from uncovering, undressing, and even from getting one hand cold. The state is worse after eating lunch. It is better from bending the head backward. (Compare with *Bryonia* and *Spongia*.) The child can be very irritable and angry.

- *Pulsatilla nigricans*. The child has all the typical symptoms of this remedy. In other words, he needs attention and is weepy and may become more tearful or just have tears flowing during the episode of cough. The cough is worse during the evening and in bed at night. It is made much better by fresh air and from lying high on a few pillows. The cough can be dry in the evening and loose in the morning. (Compare with *Hepar sulphur*.)

Diarrhea

Because treatments are available, children in civilized countries are safe in cases of acute diarrhea. But children in developing countries, who don't have access to good health care, die from this ailment by the thousands every year. The main danger posed by diarrhea is dehydration.

If your child has diarrhea, you have to make sure that he is kept well hydrated with any kind of liquid but preferably one with electrolytes such as sodium and potassium. The warning signs of dehydration are dry tongue; loose, old-looking skin; very infrequent urination; and significant weakness. If any of these signs appear in your child, you must call 9-1-1 or go to the emergency room. You should also contact a physician in any case of diarrhea that doesn't go away in a few hours after giving a remedy, even if the child seems fine.

Certainly, if your child develops diarrhea during or after a trip to one of the Third World countries, visiting a doctor is a must. You need to make sure that there's no infection. Some cases of flu have diarrhea as their main symptom. Homeopathy does miracles for that state. As a matter of fact, Jennifer Jacobs, M.D., a past president of the AIH, published a series of research papers that clearly show that homeopathy is effective for the treatment of diarrhea.

There are many remedies that can be helpful for diarrhea. I'll name only two for your home use. If diarrhea persists for more than twenty-four hours, contact your doctor.

Please be mindful that an isolated episode of liquid stools after eating too many prunes shouldn't trigger an emergency response.

- *Arsenicum album*. This remedy should always come to your mind first in cases when you suspect food poisoning. It's also extremely helpful when a child overeats or eats too much fruit and then develops diarrhea. In addition, it's frequently indicated in cases of the "stomach flu."

The child is restless, anxious, and weak and fears serious illness—even death. There's often a combination of diarrhea and vomiting. Symptoms are much worse after midnight. The stool is irritating, burning. The child feels better from warm applications to the stomach and is thirsty for small sips of cold water.

- *Veratrum album*. In my experience, this remedy is indicated in cases of stomach flu as frequently as *Arsenicum*. But whereas the emotional focus of children who need *Arsenicum* is restless anxiety, the most characteristic feature of *Veratrum* is prostration (extreme weakness and inability to move). Often the first symptom of this state is forceful vomiting accompanied by diarrhea. Sometimes the diarrhea and vomiting come simultaneously.

The child has cold sweat on the forehead and is extremely weak. The stool is profuse and odorless. The forehead and stomach are cold. If the child asks for ice cubes or salty things, or even salt, it confirms the choice of this remedy.

Earache

This is a big topic in many popular homeopathic books. The main issue here is that conventional doctors used to prescribe antibiotics for almost every case of earache. Earache usually signals the inflammation of the middle ear, which is called acute otitis media (AOM). The potential danger is that if the inflammation is left untreated, the infection can develop into meningitis (inflammation of the membranes that cover the brain and the spinal cord).

Recently, physicians have increasingly accepted the tactic of watchful waiting. If the child doesn't show obvious signs of severe infection, the doctor doesn't prescribe an antibiotic right away. Research has shown that a large proportion of cases of AOM (over 80 percent) resolve spontaneously in twenty-four to forty-eight hours. However, many parents want antibiotics for their children and believe that this treatment is necessary for ear infections. This opinion is not supported by research.

Some physicians offer parents a safety-net antibiotic prescription (SNAP). According to this method, parents get a prescription but don't fill it unless the child's condition gets worse or symptoms persist for more than one to two days. This method was investigated in a multicenter pediatric study in Cincinnati, Ohio. Of the 175 families who got a SNAP, 120 (69 percent) didn't fill the prescription, and 117 said they were willing to use pain medications without antibiotics in the future. Of the 55 families who did fill the prescription, 33 filled it within forty-eight hours of diagnosis. A large proportion of these parents cited their child's continued pain or fever as the reason.

Some countries have also adopted this policy with very good results. For example, the Netherlands already has a national policy of supportive treatment only, and using antibiotics or myringotomy (a procedure of inserting a tube in the ear to provide drainage) for less than 5 percent of diagnosed cases of AOM. In that country, a study showed that more than 90 percent of nearly five thousand children recovered from earache within a few days.

Homeopathy offers excellent remedies that provide fast relief of pain and fever. Still, you should ensure that a physician sees your child with an earache. If you give a remedy to your child on the way to the doctor, and your doctor cannot see any problems with the middle ear during the examination—fine.

If you are able to catch a first occurrence of AOM with a correct remedy, chances are that the condition won't come back for a long time. Please remember, however, that repeated ear infections require constitutional treatment by a homeopath.

A baby with an ear infection will most definitely let you know that there's a problem. The infant tosses the head around and pulls on the ear that hurts. Some crying and loud screaming is usually present, too. A correctly prescribed remedy takes care of this acute problem in a matter of minutes or, at maximum, hours.

- *Belladonna*. Use this remedy for sudden onset of a right-sided earache. The child has a very high fever, glassy eyes, and enlarged pupils.
- *Chamomilla*. The child is screaming from pain but won't allow you to touch the ear. She's also very irritable and demanding, even capricious (that is, she'll ask for something but refuse it the moment it is offered). The only thing that calms the child down is being carried. If you put the child down for even a second, the entire neighborhood will know about it right away. In other words, you have a little tyrant on your hands.

I frequently have prescribed this remedy on the phone after hearing the child screaming on the other end of the line. I always suggest to the parent, "Pick up your child so we can talk." If that works, the remedy is usually clear. Believe me, you cannot miss the indications for this remedy.

- *Ferrum phosphoricum*. This remedy is one of the most useful in the beginning of an earache, when you clearly see that there's a problem, but it doesn't look like any remedy you know. The picture is similar to *Belladonna* but doesn't fit exactly, especially in the level of intensity. It just doesn't present the clear picture that a child who needs *Belladonna* usually presents. The pain is usually on the right side.
- *Hepar sulphur*. The child is extremely sensitive to the slightest interference. For example, a cold draft (even uncovering a part of a body) or a touch can make the pain a hundred times worse. The child quickly flies into a rage. It's a different picture from *Chamomilla*. The child who needs *Chamomilla* is restless and angry

but calms down if constantly carried around. The *Hepar* child just doesn't want to be bothered with. Period.

• *Pulsatilla nigricans.* This is the most frequently required remedy in cases when otitis comes after the child first has a "cold," with yellowish-greenish nasal discharge. Then the earache begins. The child is weepy and needs affection. Symptoms are made better by fresh air and from being gently carried. It's very different from the *Chamomilla* state. Here the child is sweet and looks defenseless.

If your best choice didn't bring any relief, call the homeopath. Most probably there is an alternative to what you gave. As I said before, there are other helpful remedies, too, but finding them is more complicated and should be left to homeopaths.

Motion Sickness

What a dreadful problem motion sickness can be! I suffered from this ailment when I was a child and still have pretty significant seasickness. I'll only tell you about the two most frequently required remedies. One of them fits me very well, so I definitely know what I'm talking about firsthand.

• *Cocculus indicus.* Even watching moving objects makes a person nauseous and dizzy. Vertigo is a very important part of the child's complaints. Food odors make matters significantly worse.

• *Tabacum.* The picture is of deathly nausea. The feeling is literally that if the trip (by boat, plane, or car) continues one more minute, you'll die. The child appears so pale that sometimes the face may look green. The child is about to faint and asks to open the window of the car. Open air brings enormous relief!

By the way, isn't it funny that the pirates and salty old seamen in the movies smoke pipes? In the old days, sailors must have used a crude preparation of *Tabacum* to prevent and cure seasickness. Obviously, a homeopathic preparation offers the same benefits— minus all the dangerous complications of smoking.

Nausea and Vomiting

Nausea and vomiting are always symptoms of a more complicated problem, like motion sickness. Whenever your child develops these symptoms, you need to get your doctor involved. Here are a few common reasons they arise.

These symptoms could be side effects of a conventional medication. Sadly, a number of children have to undergo chemotherapy. Nausea is one of its major complications. Homeopathy can help in this situation.

Fortunately, there's also a simple reason for nausea: overeating. It would be nice to make sure that people never overeat, but it's unrealistic, especially on Thanksgiving, Christmas, and other holidays.

Some children have a tendency to eat indigestible items. This can cause vomiting, especially in relatively healthy children whose bodies still have a capacity to reject what is wrong. Teenagers are known to experiment with tobacco, drugs, and alcohol. These substances also cause nausea and vomiting.

- *Aethusa cynapium.* This is almost a specific for babies who vomit large curds of milk after each feeding. In this picture, the baby is not thirsty. Often the baby also has diarrhea, is weak and exhausted, and doesn't sleep well (things you'd expect from a hungry baby). I've seen numerous cases when one dose of *Aethusa* 30C changes things pretty dramatically.
- *Antimonium crudum.* Use *Antimonium* for vomiting from overeating, or eating indigestible things. The person vomits immediately after eating or drinking. The tongue has a white coating.
- *Antimonium tartaricum.* This remedy is indicated when the child vomits during coughing. Another frequent scenario is eating that results in a cough, which ends up with burping and vomiting.
- *Arsenicum album.* This remedy is used for vomiting that's a result of food poisoning. The child experiences fear when vomiting and tries not to vomit because the process causes so much fear. The overall picture will be an anxious, very chilly child who is thirsty for small sips of water. This vomiting is accompanied by burning

pains in the stomach. The vomit is acidic and irritating. If vomiting continues, the child becomes exhausted. Sometimes diarrhea goes together with vomiting. Symptoms are made much worse by cold drinks and much better by warm drinks. (Compare with *Veratrum Album*.)

• *Ipecacuanha*. *Ipecacuanha* is used for terrible nausea that isn't relieved even by vomiting. Nothing makes it better. Amazingly, the tongue remains clean. (It is a common finding in digestive disorders for the tongue to be coated.)

I find this remedy to be very helpful for people who develop nausea as a side effect of chemotherapy. In these cases, it has to be used in 6C potency. (Take three pellets, two to three times a day for the duration of chemotherapy.)

• *Nux vomica*. Infants who respond well to this remedy are well characterized by a famous American homeopath, Dr. Panos, as, "Wants to and can't." The child wants to vomit but can't. Frequently, nausea accompanies constipation when there are unsuccessful attempts to move the bowels. As you can easily imagine, the person is very irritable, sensitive to noises and bright light. Symptoms are made better by lying down and having warm drinks.

When your child grows up and starts drinking alcohol, *Nux vomica* becomes helpful for hangovers. In the case of a hangover with symptoms of irritability and increased sensitivity to noise and light, a dose of 30C can be repeated a few times. I know that teens aren't supposed to drink at college. But they do. Besides, to parents, a forty-year-old child is still a child. Teenagers (and adults) who stay up all night and feel irritable, hypersensitive, and tired in the morning would also benefit from a dose of *Nux vomica*.

• *Phosphorus*. Adolph Lippe, a famous nineteenth-century American homeopath, described an important symptom of this remedy: the person is very thirsty for cold water but vomits the moment the water warms up in the stomach. This remedy is helpful if the child vomits blood. Obviously, you'll be giving the child a dose of this remedy right after you've called 9-1-1, or on your way to the emergency room!

• *Veratrum album*. *Veratrum* is used for severe, frequent, and exhausting projectile vomiting. Often the vomiting occurs simultaneously with diarrhea. The child becomes quickly exhausted and is chilly; there's cold perspiration on the forehead. It looks like the child is about to collapse, and in some cases he may collapse. Prior to that, the child has cold breath. Symptoms worsen from drinking. (Compare with *Arsenicum*—a prominent picture of anxiety and irritating discharges, better from warm drinks, and with *Phosphorus*—not as exhausted; to the contrary, the child might remain active despite vomiting. Better from cold drinks and from lying on the right side.)

Poison Ivy

Washington Homeopathic Products, one of the oldest homeopathic companies in the United States, makes a remedy marketed under the brand name Poison Ivy Pills. This is another rare example of a proprietary product containing a single homeopathic preparation, *Rhus toxicodendron* 4X. Registered with the FDA since 1938, this product is often successful in treating poison ivy rashes. The company also recommends it for the prevention of the effects of poison ivy for people who live and work in areas rich with this plant. I cannot comment on the success of the prophylaxis, but I have recommended this product to many people for the treatment of early stages of poison ivy with great success.

Rhus tox is the main, but not the only, remedy for poison ivy and poison oak. But other remedies have fine distinctions that make their pictures difficult for a layperson to distinguish from *Rhus tox*. For example, there is a remedy, *Anacardium*, made from marking nut, which is a close relative of poison ivy. Probably only an experienced homeopath would be able to distinguish between its symptoms and those of *Rhus tox*.

A major characteristic of rashes that respond to *Rhus tox* is that the itching feels much better from a very hot shower or using any other application of scalding hot water. In this picture, the child is anxious and restless.

Two other remedies that you might be able to distinguish are the following:

- *Ledum palustre*. The child has a unique characteristic of getting better from ice-cold applications.
- *Sulphur*. Symptoms are much worse at night, especially when the child becomes heated in bed. It feels worse from any kind of heat.

If in doubt, give *Rhus tox*. In my experience (and I've had some painful experiences with poison ivy), this remedy is frequently indicated. Poison Ivy Pills are great, because their low potency doesn't cause significant aggravations. Usually, a few doses either take care of the problem or do nothing, and then you know to move on. If nothing happens soon, call a homeopath or seek other types of professional help. Rashes are uncomfortable, but they are rarely dangerous. If already under the regular care of a homeopath, the patient's constitutional remedy may work better than any of the remedies more commonly used for poison ivy.

Sinusitis (Acute)

Please understand clearly that although the remedies described in this section can be very helpful in eliminating the symptoms of acute sinusitis, and even in preventing its reoccurrence, they only will be of marginal help to children with recurring (chronic) sinus infections. Treatment of chronic sinusitis is one of the very well-known fortes of homeopathy. But it has to be done by a homeopath. You also have to make sure that you don't wait too long and so miss a point when professional help (sometimes including antibiotics) is indicated.

Making this determination is actually pretty simple. After a correct homeopathic remedy, the symptoms of acute sinusitis should get significantly better in less than six hours. If improvement doesn't happen, the next step is bringing your child to a health care professional.

- *Hydrastis canadensis.* This is indicated when nasal discharge is copious and thick. An important characteristic is a marked postnasal drip, frequently with a sore throat. People who need it usually are constipated. (Compare it with *Kali bichromicum*, but notice that those who need *Kali* frequently have deep "nasal" voices and complain of diarrhea.)
- *Kali bichromicum.* This remedy is indicated for acute sinusitis significantly more often than *Hydrastis*. It's a remedy for acute sinusitis when there is a gluey, sticky, thick greenish-yellow discharge from the nose, and someone's voice sounds nasal. In this picture, there's also a significant heaviness and burning pain at the root of the nose. There might also be a headache (characteristically in one small spot) and photophobia, or light sensitivity. If there is any problem with the stools, it's usually diarrhea. (Compare with *Hydrastis canadensis.*)
- *Mercurius solubilis.* Also a frequently indicated remedy, but unlike in the cases of *Kali* and *Hydrastis*, the green discharge flows easily and doesn't create long strings of mucus coming out of the nose. In this picture, the child has offensive breath and often tooth imprints on a coated, dirty-looking tongue. There is also drooling. You can easily detect this symptom if you see wet spots on the pillow in the morning. Another characteristic symptom is sinus pain that also radiates to the teeth.
- *Mercurius iodatus flavus* is indicated if the symptoms are strongly presented on the right side.
- *Mercurius iodatus ruber* is indicated for prominent left-sided symptoms. If there is no pronounced "sidedness" of the symptoms, use *Mercurius solubilis*.

Sore Throat

A sore throat can be one of the most frustrating issues that parents and physicians have to face. Physicians are aware of and parents are scared of strep throat with good reason. Streptococcal infections can have dangerous complications, including rheumatic fever, with the potential development of heart disease and inflammation of the kidneys.

The treatment of sore throat is a definite forte of homeopathy. After all, the first famous success that Hahnemann had was in the treatment of scarlet fever, a severe form of strep throat that we rarely see anymore. Still, you definitely want your children to be safe. You therefore should bring them to your physician so a throat culture can be taken. In many cases, sore throats are not bacterial and therefore do not require antibiotics.

According to current guidelines that physicians follow, positive results of a throat culture should always lead to the administration of antibiotics. However, the routine prescribing of antibiotics over the phone every time parents call in to say that their children are sick is bad medicine.

Homeopathy should come into play in the following situations:

1. Your child is at the very beginning of an illness when you witness the first symptoms of a cold. Using a correct remedy then will stop any further development of a sore throat. You may also want to use homeopathy if you've made an appointment with a doctor but have an hour or more to wait until the doctor can see you. Using a correct homeopathic remedy may result in a significant decrease or total elimination of symptoms, including fever and pain, prior to the appointment. Of course, this leads to a very nice, easy visit with no further treatment required.

2. You saw a physician and the throat culture came back negative. Or the physician didn't see the need to do a culture because there was no evidence of strep throat at all. Now you feel it is safe to use homeopathic remedies.

3. Your child has frequent episodes of sore throat that require antibiotics. Seize a window of opportunity when your child is between episodes to see a homeopath for constitutional treatment. Homeopathic intervention can stop the recurrence of sore throats. In some cases, the child might develop another sore throat with strong, acute symptoms. If an aggravation like this does occur, an antibiotic will work very rapidly, and then no more sore throats will be present.

Just remember, you need to consult with your doctor in all cases of sore throats. Better safe than sorry. Many remedies may be indicated in the treatment of the sore throat. I've found that the following ones are indicated most frequently:

- *Aconitum napellus*. Use this remedy for the sudden beginning of a sore throat after your child was exposed to cold, windy weather. The symptoms are very severe, and the child is scared and restless. The child is thirsty for cold drinks that are painful to swallow.
- *Belladonna*. This remedy is an absolute champion of treatment of acute sore throats. Use when the pain and burning are on the right side. The child cannot tolerate even a slight touch of the throat. Symptoms feel worse when moving the head or swallowing liquids. This picture includes high fever with a red face, large pupils, hot head, and cold hands and feet. The child may be confused.
- *Bryonia alba*. The beginning of the illness comes on slower than in a *Belladonna* state, but the fever can be rather high. Pain is made worse by any movement, even speaking. The child wants to be quiet and be left alone. The child is very thirsty.
- *Ferrum phosphoricum*. Use this for sore throat with high fever, significant weakness, but no symptoms that point to any other remedy you know.
- *Mercurius iodatus flavus*. Use this for right-sided sore throats. This state begins slower than cases that require *Belladonna*. There's offensive breath and a dirty-looking, coated tongue. It's much worse at night and with empty swallowing.

- *Mercurius iodatus ruber*. This remedy is very frequently indicated for left-sided sore throat. All other symptoms are similar to *Mercurius iodatus flavus*.

- *Phytolacca*. Use *Phytolacca* when the throat is burning. Symptoms are made much worse by hot drinks and much better by cold drinks. The glands on the neck are frequently enlarged and painful.

Teething

Anybody who has had a teething child knows how painful this experience is for both child and parent. Very few children have it easy, but I've met some who have. Remedies that are helpful can be divided into the following two categories:

1. *Remedies for acute help with pain*. We will discuss two major remedies from this group in this section: *Chamomilla* and *Belladonna*.

2. *Remedies that make the whole process easy and help in the formation of good-quality teeth*. Good baby teeth are as important as good permanent teeth. These remedies have to be prescribed by a homeopath.

There are many homeopathic combination remedies for teething babies. Some are packaged in sophisticated dispensing systems that contain prediluted remedies. The two remedies that we're going to discuss here are always included in the mix, along with one or two more remedies that are considered to be potentially helpful. I've heard many good reports from parents about these products.

Combination remedies often provide very effective temporary relief. If you are the kind of person who just wants relief without the additional headaches of finding the right remedy or going to a homeopath, you can try one. Just do not overuse it.

My preferred advice is to evaluate whether or not *Chamomilla* or *Belladonna* fit the symptoms that your baby has. If the answer is yes, go ahead and use the correct single remedy. If neither fits the symptoms, you may want to consult a homeopath. A single remedy may be given repeatedly if you see an improvement, even if the symptoms then come back. I advise using the plussing method described in Chapter Two. After all, you'll have to dissolve the pill anyway so your baby can swallow it.

In this section, I have to break the alphabetical order to present the absolute champion of all the remedies for teething first.

• *Chamomilla.* I'll begin by telling you a brief story. When the Center for Health and Healing at Beth Israel Medical Center had just opened in New York City, I gave a seminar for our staff on the basic use of homeopathy for acute conditions. My most attentive student was Larry Palevsky, M.D., who is a board-certified holistic pediatrician. Because he's a very good clinician and a caring person, I always hoped that one day he would find the time to study homeopathy. He has been able to use homeopathy for acute cases and sometimes has shared details of those situations.

One time, Dr. Palevsky received a call from a concerned mother who felt that her daughter "was going through a very difficult emotional time." In the background, he could hear the baby screaming bloody murder. He'd been following her progress since she was born and she seemed pretty well adjusted, so he asked the mother, "Do you think it's possible instead that your daughter is teething?" The psychoanalytical mother was amazed by this thought. The answer was yes! One dose of *Chamomilla* 30C resolved the issues this teething baby had.

The picture of this remedy is hard to miss. The child is in severe pain, angry, screaming, and irritable. The child doesn't want to be touched or even looked at. Frequently, symptoms are worse at night. The child might throw objects that were offered by parents, who are trying to please the child. The child feels better when being constantly carried around. If in doubt, try to put your little teething devil down. You might hear everyone on your block screaming, "Pick the baby up!"

• *Belladonna*. The baby who needs this remedy won't be as cross as the one with *Chamomilla* symptoms. The key here is inflammation with confusion. The child has a flushed face, has a fever, and acts confused. In the midst of confusion, the baby might strike out or (frequently) bite. Don't take it personally. Just give a dose of *Belladonna* 30C.

Chapter Seven will give you instructions for using these remedies to assist you in improving your own child's health and well-being.

Chapter Seven

Instructions for Using Homeopathic Remedies

In this chapter, you'll find all the strategic information necessary to help your children fight and win their battles with acute ailments. For mild acute conditions and emergencies, you should always try to give your child a remedy as soon as possible. As a parent, you need to seize the opportunity to help your child in the first few minutes or hours of the illness. You also need to know what to do for first aid and in acute situations, in which you'll serve as your child's first-response team. For serious acute conditions, it's always best to seek help from a homeopath as soon as you can.

Most important, this chapter will help you understand how to interpret the information about remedies found in the last chapter. You may now know a remedy is helpful for symptoms on the left side of the body or that it's for someone who feels better when lying down, but what is the significance of such facts? Why do they matter? You'll find out later in the chapter, in the section called "Choosing the Right Homeopathic Remedy for Your Child."

What You Can Do in an Emergency

Even if you have to take your child to the emergency room, giving your child an appropriate homeopathic remedy on the way there may save both your child—and you—from a lot of grief. There have been numerous cases when a child gets completely better after taking a remedy and walks away from the ER without anything additional needing to be done. Take the following example from my younger daughter's life.

When she was ten, my daughter's uncle and her sixteen-year-old cousin came to visit. They gave my daughter a beautiful bicycle as a present. Excited, the two cousins immediately decided to take it out for a spin. Although we didn't have a helmet for her yet, my daughter pleaded with my wife and me to let her ride it. "The bike is so cute! Why can't we go just a few blocks and come back? Please, please, *pleeease!*" Finally, they were granted permission to travel a few blocks on a quiet street near our house. My daughter was riding the bike; her cousin was skating alongside on roller blades.

The girls were so excited about getting together that they weren't watching as carefully as they should have, and they failed to notice a neighbor parking her car in her driveway. My daughter was hit and knocked over by the woman's slow-moving car. The surprised driver was scared by the accident. She jumped out of her car, rushed to my daughter's side, and phoned 9-1-1. She did all she could. My niece called my wife.

My daughter didn't think there was a problem. Although her head had hit the pavement and she was in pain, she wanted to continue riding her new bike. Instead she was taken to the ER of the local hospital. My wife followed behind the ambulance and called me from her car phone. Based on our daughter's symptoms, I suggested giving her a pellet of *Arnica montana* 200C as soon as possible. My daughter received the remedy on arrival. Then she also had a complete medical workup, which included a CAT scan of her brain to rule out bleeding. Everything was normal. She came home in a few hours.

Better safe than sorry! If your child's condition has the potential to be serious, please call your doctor or go to the emergency room. You can always give your child a homeopathic remedy on the way there. In many cases, the remedy will take care of your child's problem before you even get to meet the doctor—and that's OK, because the improvement isn't an illusion. The doctor can confirm that any danger has passed.

You needn't worry that you'll harm your child by making a mistake in selecting a remedy, so long as you go to the doctor or ER when conditions warrant it and don't hand out extra doses. Earlier in the book, we discussed reasons why multiple doses aren't advisable: they can cause provings. But a single dose of a wrong remedy has no impact. A little bit later in this chapter, you'll learn how to choose the right remedy.

An important beneficial feature of homeopathy is that it doesn't mask serious problems. A conventional painkiller may forcefully block pain, yet the problem causing the pain in the first place remains untreated. Pain exists to alert us to danger and injury. Homeopathic remedies work by addressing underlying issues, such as those that might cause pain, on a deep, systemic level. But remedies don't suppress the pain response. If a remedy is wrong for your child's particular condition, or if a homeopathic remedy cannot resolve the problem, your child's symptoms will remain unchanged, and the doctor won't miss important symptoms of the illness.

To Treat or Not to Treat—That Is the Question

There are as many possible scenarios that you could face as there are children in the world. But if one of your main goals is to raise kids who stand good chances of becoming strong, healthy adults, then you must learn when to offer your children medication and when to let them heal on their own.

If I had to name a single factor that is responsible for the overuse of any medications in treating children, I'd definitely name parents as that cause. The most important piece of advice for parents who want to improve the overall health of their offspring is to have children stay at home when they're feeling sick. Resorting to suppressive medication is a strategy often aimed at keeping the wheels of life turning. After all, adults need to go to work and children need an education. Sometimes a day off is not an option.

Allowing sick children the space and time to heal is a strategy that creates a more favorable environment for healing. Homeopathic remedies give the body a push, but the body does the job of healing. For the body to do a better job, it needs optimal conditions. Staying home to rest means children aren't distracted by a need to handle other stressors, which might include exposure to additional bacteria and viruses, noise, physical activity, the need to pay attention, and demands from teachers and other students.

Think about it. Your nine-year-old daughter wakes up feeling not too good and she has the sniffles. You take her temperature. It's 98.6 degrees Fahrenheit. "No fever, she has to go to school," you decide. So you give her some cold medicine that contains decongestant and antihistamine ingredients, and you put her on the bus. Not a good idea!

Your child is getting sick. Even if your child is a total genius and goes to a school where every teacher is an Einstein, she can easily skip a few days. Give her some rest, some love, some chicken soup. Recent studies have shown that these ordinary things—including the chicken soup—help the immune system to fight illness.

On top of that, you could give your child a single dose of a homeopathic remedy. But I definitely wouldn't reach for a bottle of conventional cold medicine just yet. Don't you agree that maybe, just maybe, if parents took the steps listed here instead of sending sick and medicated children to school, those children wouldn't get sick all the time?

We have to provide children with an environment that's optimal for growing healthy. One or two days at home when they're just coming down with a cold can save them a lot of future trouble, because it gives them a chance to strengthen their defense mechanisms. Then the next time a virus comes along, children won't even notice it.

A medication of any type, including homeopathy, isn't always the answer! Parents frequently report to me with great pride, "I give my son *Arnica* every time he falls!" or, "We give our daughter *Oscillococcinum* every time there's a cold or a flu going around at school!" Again, sending them to school is not a good idea, despite that they're using homeopathy.

Appropriate treatment is indicated by the severity of an illness. Minor ailments, such as bumps and bruises from falling on the playground, usually don't require any intervention or require only supportive measures. There's no reason to fire a cannon at a fly. Children have enormous capacity to heal, especially from everyday ailments. You can always apply some *Arnica* cream or lotion on a bruise—*except if the skin is broken*—but there's truly no reason to medicate an otherwise healthy child. Of course, if your child takes a hard fall and looks shaken, a dose of *Arnica* 200C is strongly indicated even if he tells you that everything is fine when you approach him.

As a rule of thumb, minor problems that don't require a homeopathic remedy are those that have no systemic impact on a person. Serious problems that do require immediate attention can be recognized because they usually affect the whole person, meaning on the multiple levels of body, mind, and emotions.

Here are some examples to illustrate this distinction. Little Rosie is horsing around with her dad and falls. When she stands up and starts to cry, her father notices a tiny bump on Rosie's arm. "My poor little baby," says Dad. He picks up his daughter, hugs and kisses her, and she stops crying and starts to run around again.

Is there a need for any medication? Not really. If this kind of accident happens to your child, you're to put ointment on the bump if you feel you absolutely must do something. Otherwise there's just going to be a black-and-blue mark on your child's arm that will go away in a few days.

A week later, Rosie has some playmates over. Little Bobby is so excited that he can't resist pushing Rosie. He pushes her so hard that she falls on the floor and hits her head. Now she's scared. Her mouth opens for a cry, but nothing comes out for a few moments. Then she starts to sob and can't stop for a long time. Rosie wants her mother to pick her up and hold her. Even then, tears are pouring down her cheeks.

After pushing Rosie, Bobby keeps going and hits their playmate Pete so hard that he also falls down. Pete looks pale, he is obviously in pain, but he says, "I'm OK. I don't need anything."

On this occasion, at least two of the children require treatment. Rosie is scared, indicating she was affected systemically. She developed symptoms that create a picture of a state treatable with the homeopathic remedy *Pulsatilla*. In contrast, Pete presents with a typical picture of *Arnica montana*. Furthermore, if Bobby has a tendency to be violent with other children, his parents might want to consult a homeopath. Whereas Rosie and Pete need treatment for acute conditions, Bobby might benefit from constitutional treatment for his emotions, which will be described in Part Three.

Please, if your knee-jerk response is to give a homeopathic remedy to your child for everyday occurrences, next time assess the situation before you do. Maybe it's really a benign issue that doesn't require any treatment. Your child needs to be able to deal with simple situations without unnecessary help. My mother told me that she used to bring me to see a doctor for every minor problem. Clearly, it wasn't *my* problem that was being treated by the doctor; it was *her* problem. Fortunately, she didn't give me unnecessary drugs that would weaken my resilience.

Giving your children superfluous treatment, even if it's homeopathy, can be harmful to them. True, with homeopathy, one dose of a remedy isn't dangerous. Nonetheless repeated administration of various remedies one after the other isn't healthy. For instance, imagine your son has a high fever. You decide to give him *Belladonna*. It doesn't work. So you give him another remedy, and then another, and then another. Finally, your son is doing much worse than he was before any remedies were given.

If someone continues taking even a correctly prescribed remedy too frequently, a proving may happen. This means the recipient of the remedy will feel a worsening of the symptoms and could develop new symptoms. So please do not give remedies frequently and do not give one remedy after the other if you don't see an effect.

If the first remedy doesn't work, you can always go back and analyze your child's symptoms again. If you see where a mistake was made and can clearly understand what remedy actually has to be given, the administration of *one dose* of this new remedy is fine. But stop if homeopathy doesn't work on the second try. Also go back and review "Four Guidelines for Coordinating Your Child's Health Care" in Chapter Two.

But I need to reiterate this: don't give any remedies unless they are clearly indicated! If you're sure you clearly see the symptoms dictating a particular remedy, give the remedy once.

It's important to understand your own parenting style. Some people take things too easy. They do nothing, or very little, even when the situation requires prompt, aggressive treatment. Real emergencies must be treated as such each and every time. If you don't have the ability to recognize a crisis, or you generally brush off complaints and hope for the best, consider making a decision now to be more proactive or deliberate. What if the problem was more serious than you originally thought?

There are many situations when the first person on the scene, so to speak, is a parent. Knowing what remedy to give in the first hours, or sometimes minutes, of the acute illness or the accident may save you a lot of trouble in the future. Just remember that you aren't a doctor and should always err on the side of caution. Seek help.

Choosing the Right Homeopathic Remedy for Your Child

Now, if you were choosing a conventional medication instead of homeopathy, all you'd need would be the name of the condition, for instance *fever* or *sore throat*. You would pick up a package at the drugstore that says, "for fever" on the label. Seems simple.

But that isn't the way homeopathic remedies are chosen. The name of the condition is almost irrelevant. Homeopaths take disease names into account only because they help us know which of the characteristics we're seeing in a child are individual and which are universal. Whereas sore throat would be a universal condition, "left-sided sore throat" would be an individual and informative characteristic we could work with. At first, this may seem tricky, and possibly confusing, but it's true.

As you set out to explore this strange new form of medicine, I can imagine how you might be feeling: "This guy has told me about all sorts of complicated rules and theories, and now he expects me just to start giving the remedies to my children. But homeopathy is so difficult that even regular doctors can't figure it out!"

Wrong! The beauty of homeopathy is that in emergencies and acute situations, the body always tries to externalize the illness and does so with a lot of energy. That's why symptoms of an acute condition usually are obvious—easy to recognize—and easy to treat. *You can do it!* Everyone can choose the right remedy. Doctors, too, if they want to! (Many allopathic physicians were taught that homeopathy *couldn't* work, so they haven't bothered trying.) Try homeopathy and you'll see how quickly and gently it works.

In order to choose the correct homeopathic remedy for your child, you'll need to stick to a few basics. To begin with, above all else, be calm. Important decisions of every kind, and especially about what remedy to use, must be made with a cool head. If you've got a tendency to panic in an emergency, you won't be of much use to your family, as they'll have to make sure *you're* OK before handling other matters. You might even consider seeking constitutional homeopathic treatment. By the way, I've seen plenty of fathers become hysterical and mothers who were the strong ones. Ideally, at least one parent in your household can stay calm.

Second, don't play doctor. If you feel that you're in over your head with homeopathy, seek professional help. Visiting a homeopath is the best way to handle confusion. Even a brief phone consultation can often clarify an issue and provide a solution to the question of what remedy to give your child.

If you don't have access to a good local homeopath, call your physician or go to the nearest ER. The safety of your child comes first. You aren't expected to know it all. Next time, you'll do better.

Third, remember to keep an open mind. We all tend to look for what we know, and most of us share the desire to adjust reality to our wishes. That's why people who only know a few remedies typically look for signs indicating the need for these remedies. Trouble is, they'll always find them, even if they aren't there!

Taking all of this into account, here are the steps to follow:

1. *First look at the big picture*. No matter what the problem is, there's always more than one symptom involved. Frequently, one of the few major homeopathic remedies is indicated. As discussed earlier in the book, remedies that have many widespread uses and cover a wide variety of mental, emotional, and physical problems are called *polychrests*. These remedies have very prominent characteristics. When you can see characteristics of a polychrest in your sick child, give it *regardless* of what specific ailment your child has.

- Give it if you notice significant changes in the way your child behaves, such as in mood, appetite, thirst.

- Give it if symptoms are worse or better at the particular time of the day or night, from heat or cold, in a warm room or outside, from assuming a specific position, or from movement or being still.

- Give it if there are new prominent fears or other emotional features. These are the most important symptoms of any. In homeopathic parlance, they're called *mentals* and *generals*.

Let's say a bee stung your son. A very specific and frequently indicated remedy for bee stings, as you'll recall from Chapter Six, is *Apis mellifica*. But it's not the right remedy for everyone who gets stung. Remember, in homeopathy we treat people, rather than the names of conditions. In this case, something else proves better. When you're watching your son, you see that he's extremely scared, restless, and agitated. He has an expression of horror on his face. This is a picture of *Aconitum napellus*. If you see these particular signs clearly, that's actually going to be the remedy of choice.

Or let's say your son is developing a cold with a high fever after receiving a vaccination. You look through the list of remedies corresponding to colds and flu that are mentioned in this book and find a few that have very clear indications. But none of them fits your son's case. He is very irritable and angry. His face is red and swollen. And he is screaming like a lunatic. Well, surprise, surprise, this is a picture of *Apis*, even though there was no bee sting involved in your son's acute condition. So give that remedy to the boy. He will get better.

2. *If you can't see significant changes in the big picture, look for local indications.* Sometimes all that's there are local changes. Then you have to note what side of the body is worse and what kind of pain the child is experiencing. An older child or teenager probably can make distinctions like these. But don't question young children about the location and the character of their pain too much. It's difficult for small children to distinguish, and there are many other symptoms to go by. You'll be able to find them both in your child and in the descriptions of remedies in this book.

3. *Choose the remedy based on what your child has, not on what the child doesn't have.* If all the signs your child is exhibiting indicate *Belladonna*, but there's no coldness of the hands or feet, it's still OK to give your child this remedy. Few people develop every symptom of a particular remedy. But it's hard to imagine giving *Aconitum* to someone who is calm and whose symptoms developed gradually. As you read the list of potential remedies in Chapter Six, the features necessary for you to make a confident choice will be clearly explained.

4. *Think in a simple way.* A wise man once said, "When you hear hooves, think of horses, not zebras." Don't fantasize about the deeper meaning of symptoms. Just go with the instinct that's coming to you. High fever, red-hot face, enlarged pupils, confused? Most probably the child needs *Belladonna*. Stung by a bee? The area is swollen, red, and painful, and the child is irritable? *Apis*. See how easy it is?

To identify symptoms, ask the following series of questions:

1. *Where is the problem?* No matter how ridiculous this sounds, you need to be clear on where the main focus of the illness is. Otherwise you'll have to consider too many remedies—unless you get lucky and the illness presents with a clear picture of one of the most common "big" remedies. For instance, in cases of trauma, if the damage is done mostly to the fingers, you'll think about *Hypericum*. If it's an eyeball that's damaged, you'll consider *Symphytum*.

2. *What changes have been brought about by the illness?* For example, if your child used to be thirsty and now, with the onset of fever, he is not thirsty, that's an important symptom. It's a definite change. If the main presentation of the flu in your child is aching pains, your choices will boil down to *Eupatorium* or *Bryonia*. If the main presentation is weakness, you'll first think about *Gelsemium*. If the main presentation is hypersensitivity to all stimuli, you'll first consider *Nux vomica*.

The answer "He is thirsty for ice-cold water" carries important information for a homeopath, whereas "He likes Coke but hates Mountain Dew" means nothing, because it is an ongoing personal preference.

3. *How quickly did the symptoms develop?* Seconds, days, weeks, months, or even years are all legitimate answers.

4. *What makes symptoms better or worse?* The answer "His temperature is made better from Tylenol" contains no useful information for a homeopath, whereas "Her cough is much worse when she lies down" is a major homeopathic treasure. Known in homeopathy as *modalities*, details that reflect *when* and *what* make symptoms better or worse always refer to natural things, never to medications.

For a homeopath, the most useful modalities are the following:

- Temperature of the environment
- Time of day
- Environmental conditions (for example, cold, hot, dry, wet)

- Position of the body (for example, doubled over, sitting up, lying down)
- Particular activity (for example, talking, eating, drinking, moving, resting)
- Sensory reactions (for example, bright light, loud noise)
- Location in the body (for example, left side, right side, head, foot)

Just Do Your Best, Trust Yourself

It isn't a big deal if you fail to find the correct remedy. You can always fall back on conventional drugs, call your doctor, or go to the ER. Next time, you'll have more experience and will do better at identifying what's appropriate.

Of course, it's always a good idea to consult with a homeopathic practitioner. That's one of the ways you'll learn. Even when you don't have access to a homeopath right away, talking about the situation the next day with a professional may clarify what remedy should have been given. In this way—through consultations—you'll discover what to do the next time there's a similar group of symptoms.

Descriptions of various remedy pictures might seem confusing at first, because, in some cases, their differences are subtle. But don't let that stop you from making a choice. Trust yourself. With the help of this book, chances are that you'll be successful most of the time. It's designed to provide you with information you can use right away.

Chapters Eight and Nine discuss the homeopathic approach to various chronic problems. Chapter Eight explores the homeopathic approach to treating chronic mental health problems and Chapter Nine explores the homeopathic approach to treating chronic physical problems.

Part Three

Treating Chronic Mental Health and Physical Problems

Chapter Eight

Treating Chronic Mental Health Problems

The rest of the book will be dedicated to the homeopathic approach to various chronic problems. You'll read many stories of successful and often seemingly miraculous treatments with homeopathy. As you read these cases, please remember that although the process of choosing a remedy may seem simple, it is not. When presented to you on a piece of paper by an expert homeopath, after the fact, a conscious effort is made to explain the decision as simply and straightforwardly as possible, so you can appreciate the choice of the remedy. In real life, collecting and evaluating information about a child is complex. Arriving at a successful prescription requires good clinical skills and a detailed knowledge of homeopathic medications. These abilities only come after many years of study, professional mentoring, and hands-on experiences.

As with any other type of medicine, attempting to substitute your own "kitchen table homeopathy" for professional homeopathic consultation won't be effective. If you resist reaching out for help when your child is chronically ill, chances are high that you'll be disappointed, which does the child no good.

My intention in Chapters Eight and Nine is to clearly illustrate how much can be accomplished during homeopathic treatment for long-lasting and sometimes severe conditions. I hope this information will open your eyes to the elegance of the homeopathic solution.

How Homeopathy Approaches Mental Illness

Mental illness is on the rise in our children. Increasingly, they suffer from anxiety disorder, depression, bipolar disorder, ADHD, and autism. Ages ago, children suffered and died from superficial illnesses, such as infections and skin diseases. Now illness reaches our children at the core of their being, where it becomes chronic. Yes, they will probably live longer, but they are sicker and they are bound to be chronically ill. They are sicker on a deeper level. They may even need to take medications every day of their lives. What fun is it to start antidepressants at age ten and continue taking them for the rest of your life? We need to stop this trend right now. Homeopathy can help.

Constitutional care is appropriate for any type of chronic illness. Its purpose is to restore children to their natural state of health, as it was if they were born healthy. Care of chronic ailments is known as *constitutional treatment,* because the homeopath attempts to initiate a healing process of the entire child. As it is a more complicated process than identifying the correct remedy for an acute condition, this type of prescribing must be undertaken in consultation with a homeopath. Because the whole child, with all of his or her individual characteristics, must be thoroughly evaluated, only a homeopath will be able to achieve the necessary precision in selecting the right remedy.

For decades, homeopathic practitioners and theoreticians have paid close attention to the treatment of various emotional problems. Our arsenal is well stocked with remedies that can treat any type of chronic emotional or mental problem effectively. As you saw in Part One, "An Introduction to Homeopathic Treatment for Children," the direction of cure is expected to move from inside to outside. Emotional and mental problems appear at the deepest, most protected level of the human being. It's the place where our children's overall healing process needs to and can begin.

Finding and prescribing the correct homeopathic remedy brings about spectacular results in the majority of cases. But because mental illness is so deep inside our being, the process of recovery, especially from very serious problems, requires patients to be tolerant sometimes of fairly painful symptoms that can appear on more superficial levels as the healing of their minds takes place.

Healing mental illness with homeopathy becomes complicated when patients, psychologists, and physicians who are inexperienced in this approach try to reconcile methods from conventional psychiatry and general medicine with the homeopathic view of a human being. Their "common sense" notion that would dictate the use of different medications for "independent" problems simply doesn't apply here. Clear understanding of the main principles of homeopathy and strict adherence to them are the key to the success or failure of constitutional homeopathic treatment.

One can't possibly trick nature. If you hope that in your particular case the rules of homeopathy don't apply, you're wrong. If the material you read in the chapters in this part of the book seems like a repetition of what you've already learned, I'm actually elated. That means you've been paying attention and know what to do.

The Healing Crisis

Homeopathy is very clear. If a person has a significant emotional or mental problem, the remedy that's prescribed must address this core issue rather than a more peripheral complaint. Throughout the period that it takes to resolve the core issue, it's required that no interference with the ongoing treatment happen.

Unfortunately, a lot of people disregard an important point. They're enthusiastic at the beginning of treatment; however, they tend to ignore this rule, especially as they get better and move further from the initial complaint. In the process of healing, the person may experience a healing crisis in which, after the improvement of the main problem, they may undergo a brief return and cure of old complaints. There's a temptation to slip.

For the overwhelming majority of people who aren't familiar with homeopathy, noninterference can raise numerous issues. One of the most difficult parts of it is the need to tolerate whatever physical complaints may appear. For example, quite a few years ago, I saw Idis. At age fourteen, she developed a significant depression after her family moved to a new town and she was separated from her friends. That same year, both of her grandparents passed away. A sensitive and reserved person, Idis generally kept most of her feelings to herself. But in this situation, her parents began to notice that their daughter spent longer and longer hours alone and really didn't want any company. She was noticed crying loudly alone in her room. Her academic performance was also bad. Soon her concerned parents brought her to my office.

After an hour and a half of initial evaluation, the situation was clear. Idis was depressed. She wasn't suicidal and she wanted to get better, but she couldn't enjoy her life at all. I began looking for more identifying traits in her body and behavior by following the guidelines of homeopathy. Her parents told me that when Idis was six, she fell off her bike and developed significant headaches, which gradually went away. Combining that information with Idis's other characteristics led me to select the right remedy. Idis was also getting pimples. Interestingly, she volunteered that she'd begun to crave salty foods more and more. There were enough clear symptoms that indicated a homeopathic remedy, *Natrum muriaticum* (sodium chloride). On top of her isolation, weepiness, and headaches, she had a craving for salt, which was a final confirmation that this remedy would be her simillimum.

As described in Chapter Seven, in the section called "Choosing the Right Homeopathic Remedy for Your Child," we first look at the big picture. I therefore paid attention to the emotional and general changes that were characteristic to Idis. On the mental level, her changes included a depressed mood, being reserved, and refusing consolation. Generally speaking, the most remarkable features I noted were the headaches she had as a result of a trauma (her bike accident) and craving salt. The next level we look at is the level of local indications. So I also wanted to know more about the location of Idis's symptoms. Her acne, for example, appeared mostly on her forehead. This specific detail allowed me to narrow down the number of remedies I was considering to thirty-five. It also showed me that *Natrum muriaticum* was a strong possibility. In the *Repertory*, *Natrum muriaticum* is listed under this rubric—pimples on the forehead—as only one of twenty-one that are highly indicated for this condition.

Essentially, the same rules apply to finding remedies for both acute and chronic conditions. But in chronic cases, the symptoms are significantly more difficult to discern. Because chronically sick children have been ill for an extended period of time, their minds and bodies create hundreds—and sometimes thousands—of symptoms. Changes are always more significant than characteristics that have remained the same. Only an experienced homeopath can figure out which ones *are* important in choosing a remedy and which ones *aren't*. We look for changes in mood, appetite, thirst, and behavior. We look for the time of day that a symptom feels worse or better. We look at prominent fears, as well as other mental and emotional features, and at localized indications, small distinguishing features, such as on which side of the body a pain is felt.

In some cases, the picture of the right homeopathic remedy, the simillimum, becomes clear to an experienced homeopath even without cross-referencing a patient's key symptoms in the *Repertory*. The defining factor in seeing the remedy picture isn't the severity of the illness. The essential features of the selection process are the ability to see what the main problem is and what characteristic symptoms are present that are unique to a particular person. Because of my prior experience, in Idis's case I honed right in on them.

Interestingly, homeopathic remedies may be helpful for literally thousands of symptoms. *Natrum muriaticum*, for example, is known to cure thousands of symptoms. Provings done on healthy test subjects and the results of two hundred–plus experiences of using this remedy to cure thousands of people revealed these symptoms, which are listed in the *Materia Medica* and the *Repertory*. Frequently, matching a remedy to an individual patient requires laborious analysis, but in some lucky cases the majority of most characteristic symptoms of a remedy are plain to see. In homeopathic parlance, symptoms that appeared very strongly in the majority of provers are called *keynote symptoms*. When present, they lead to a very clear choice of the remedy. This was the case for Idis.

In Idis's case, the combination of her having a depressed mood, being reserved, refusing consolation, having headaches after trauma, and craving salt were all keynote symptoms strongly pointing to *Natrum muriaticum*. Her history of developing depression after the separation from her friends also strongly supported my choice of this particular remedy.

In homeopathic literature, the biblical story of Lot's wife (Gen. 19:17–26) is frequently presented as a metaphor for people who need *Natrum muriaticum*.

> The angels hastened Lot, saying, "Arise, take thy wife, and thy two daughters, which are here; lest thou be consumed in the iniquity of the city. Escape for thy life; look not behind thee, neither stay thou in all the plain; escape to the mountain, lest thou be consumed." Then the Lord rained upon Sodom and upon Gomorrah brimstone and fire from the Lord out of heaven; and he overthrew those cities, and all the plain, and all the inhabitants of the cities, and that which grew upon the ground. *But his wife looked back from behind him, and she became a pillar of salt.* [Emphasis is the author's.]

If present, this feature of constantly looking back and dwelling on losses in life, strongly points toward *Natrum muriaticum*.

I understand that the selection of this remedy might seem simple to you when you are reading my case analysis. In reality, extracting the essence of such cases is difficult and requires years of training and experience. As you already know, the requirement in homeopathic prescribing is to cure like with like—the principle of similars. So the only thing I had to do was find the right match, by answering this question: Which substance in the original provings had caused the symptoms that Idis was now exhibiting? I needed to give her a remedy that was homeopathically prepared (diluted and succussed) from that substance, which in this case was sodium chloride. If you just started reading here, or this doesn't make sense to you, please go back and reread Chapter Two. I can't impress upon you enough how central the principle of similars is to homeopathy. Remarkable, seemingly miraculous cures take place once the right remedy has been identified. Then homeopathy looks magical or too easy to be true. Nonetheless that's how well it works.

Each symptom taken alone wouldn't have indicated the choice of this remedy, *Natrum muriaticum*. What was really important was the constellation of seemingly unrelated features that Idis was presenting. Whereas a homeopathically naive person might miss the picture, an experienced homeopath would consider this particular remedy a good choice.

After studying her case and comparing the emerging picture of the remedy with pictures of other potentially helpful homeopathic medications, I gave Idis one dose of her remedy in potency 1M and told her and her parents that as her depression went away, there was a high probability that the headaches might briefly come back. But then they would disappear. I warned the parents to be prepared for numerous requests from Idis to see a dermatologist after she emerged from her depression. It was critical that they not intervene with the course of her healing process. Of course, I also advised Idis that her pimples would go away but said that they were going to be the last part of her illness to disappear. I expected the following order of events:

- Depression gets better.
- Then headaches may come back and pimples may get worse.
- Headaches go away, but pimples are still not better or are even worse.
- Then pimples go away.

All the information that I gave to Idis and her family was so new and unusual to them that she and her parents just said thank you and went home with a clear expression of doubt on their faces.

I suspected we were in for trouble. Six weeks later, a new Idis came to my office. She wasn't depressed. She wasn't isolating as much. She wasn't crying. Her school performance was better. She'd even made a new friend. (One friend for such a reserved girl means a lot!) And so far, I was wrong about everything else. Idis had no headaches. And her pimples weren't better or worse.

Cautiously, this young lady asked me whether I wanted to reconsider my previous statement about not touching the pimples. I didn't change my mind. No, ma'am! We scheduled a second follow-up appointment in eight weeks, and I clearly reminded the family to call me if any serious problems arose. No new dose was given. Things were going well.

Just a few weeks before the next appointment, Idis's mother phoned to tell me that Idis had one big headache a week before and a few small ones a few days later. They all went away pretty quickly. I was pleased to hear this information. It meant that Hering's Law was working. To me, and I hope to you by now, it meant that Idis was going through the classic healing process. Her symptoms were appearing and disappearing chronologically backward. The headaches were an indication of a brief healing crisis.

What about her pimples? Well, at the follow-up visit the pimples looked pretty "angry." Idis was desperate. She was fourteen! Being the happy father of two daughters myself, I can easily appreciate the issue. Still, Mother Nature has her own way. With all the understanding in the world, I informed Idis and her parents that I still had to advise them against antibiotics and hormone-containing creams. Idis's body was healing at the core level, and it wouldn't be appropriate to intervene.

They seemed to understand. But the difference was that this advice was written in stone in my mind, and it was written in erasable ink in their minds. Idis was persistent and in a few short weeks the happy family went to a dermatologist who had a few laughs with them about "this strange homeopath" and prescribed an antibiotic and a cream.

Two months later, beautiful Idis was back in my office with excruciating long-lasting headaches. Her mood wasn't the best in the world, which could have been a result of the headaches. Fortunately, they came back to me as soon as they did. Her remedy picture hadn't changed. Idis stopped taking conventional drugs, took her remedy again, and felt better in only a month.

Guess what. The pimples came back. But this time, Idis promised to give me a year to deal with them, and everything ultimately worked out to everyone's satisfaction.

Of course, this process of healing in reverse stages doesn't have to be present all the time. Frequently, symptoms of ADHD (or whatever else the current emotional issue may be) are all the child has ever had. In this case, we don't expect any significant problems to emerge on the physical level.

Suppression as a Potential Source of Mental Illness

Unfortunately, movement of a problem from a superficial level to a much deeper level can also happen. Please don't be too alarmed. A majority of kids successfully suppress their pimples and go happily on about their lives. But sensitive children may develop significant emotional problems as a result of persistently using a suppressive treatment, conventional or not. Here is another astonishing example from my practice.

Carmen, a seventeen-year-old girl from Argentina, was intelligent and beautiful. Her parents brought her to my office because she had developed bizarre delusions. Carmen was convinced that she was a famous assassin who went around and hurt people. All she had were thoughts, no action. And she sort of knew that. But her thoughts were so convincing that she assumed they were real. Carmen stopped going to school for fear that she might hurt or even kill somebody.

The family took Carmen to a psychologist. He was familiar with my work and recommended that the parents set up a consultation with me to see whether homeopathy could help. My secretary received their call and simply made an appointment.

Then I received a call from the psychologist. After he told me her symptoms, I began to think that Carmen was in a seriously bad situation. Her symptoms, in combination with her age, could mean the onset of schizophrenia. This worried me. Although homeopathy can be helpful for schizophrenia, often, as patients get better with homeopathy, they begin developing severe symptoms on the physical level, as Idis did in the previous story. If they wind up receiving conventional treatment at that point, it suppresses the healing process. Then the patient is back to square one.

Apparently, Carmen had developed a severe case of eczema that covered most of her arms. First, she went to a dermatologist, who prescribed some antibiotic pills and a cream. The eczema improved completely, but then Carmen started having episodes of severe anxiety and depression, and she was advised to stop the treatment.

A few months later, Carmen went to a practitioner of Chinese medicine, who gave her an herbal medicine for skin disorders. After only one dose of the herbs, Carmen developed the delusions that she came to treat in my office.

After hearing her story, I evaluated Carmen's mental status and learned that there was absolutely no family history of psychiatric illness. My understanding of the situation was that the suppressive treatment of skin eruptions in a sensitive individual (Carmen) had triggered a problem on a much deeper, emotional level. Now I had some hope.

Carmen's delusions could still be signs of the beginning of schizophrenia, triggered by repeated stress. One might guess that she'd fallen victim to a combination of a genetic predisposition to schizophrenia and significant side effects from one or both of the medications she'd taken. To me, a homeopath, the remedy picture remained the same. A sensitive individual had reacted to suppressive treatment for a strong, superficially exhibited symptom (eczema) with a disturbance on a deep emotional level.

I was willing to try homeopathy. After a long interview, I prescribed a remedy. Subsequently, I was happy to hear that Carmen got better in about two weeks. At her follow-up appointment in six weeks, I saw that a different remedy was now indicated. A dose of this new remedy brought about a very significant improvement. The improvement was such that Carmen even started talking about eczema again.

Her mother called me a few times to discuss this issue with me. We even had an appointment for me to talk to Carmen directly. Initially, she said OK, she understood. Then her eczema got so much worse that she gave her parents an ultimatum. They went to a dermatologist, who prescribed an antibiotic for Carmen and assured them that there was absolutely no danger of any psychosis being induced by the medication.

Thankfully, Carmen's mother managed to persuade her daughter to hold off taking the drug. We had a phone conversation, and I promised that the next time she came in, if I saw signs of a next remedy, one that's known to help with eczema, I would give it to her.

I hope these two real stories I've shared drive the point that I'm making all the way into your heart, not only into your brain. All that's been said in this chapter applies to the treatment of any serious emotional problem. I do appreciate the difficulties that your child may be facing as the healing process ensues. But there's no bargaining with nature. This is the way it is.

Making the Right Choice: Homeopathy Versus Allopathy

You probably expect me to say that the *expression* offered by homeopathy is always superior to the *suppression* offered by conventional drugs. Theoretically, it could be true, but the realities of modern life dictate a different and more complicated answer. You need to be aware of this issue because, as a caregiver and as a concerned parent, you'll have to make an informed choice of which way to go: homeopathy or allopathy.

First, you need to understand clearly the circumstances of your child's life. Here is an example from my practice. A few years ago, Peter was brought to my office at the Continuum Center for Health and Healing. His mother, a medical professional herself, had heard many things about my work with children and teenagers, and she was very excited to bring Peter over. She thought he was suffering from anxiety and depression. As the conventional medications offered to him hadn't really worked before, the family wanted to try "something different." Peter was fifteen. At the last moment, he had a change of plans. He told his mother that he'd come on his own and they'd meet in the waiting room.

The waiting room at the center is large and beautiful. It's very holistic. There are a few comfortable couches, many beautiful plants, and nice background music. So imagine how I felt when, after being informed by the front desk that my patient had arrived, I came out to get him and found a young man dressed like a punk rocker lying on one of the expensive sofas with all his winter clothes on, including sneakers, and his CD player was blasting. I knew because I could hear music coming out of his earphones.

Peter was half asleep. I woke him up and suggested starting our conversation right away. By the time we'd reached the door of my office, his mother also arrived. With their permission, I started my evaluation in the form of a one-to-one conversation with Peter.

I've been around the block quite a few times. Drug use came to my mind right away. Regardless of how "liberated" a person is, only someone high or drunk would be able to put on a show like he'd done in the waiting room.

Confronted with a firm, but friendly, line of questioning that also showed him my familiarity with the drug scene, Peter opened up a little bit. By the end of our twenty-minute conversation, I knew that this young man was using every substance he possibly could. For one thing, he was snorting (inhaling though the nose) the antidepressant he'd previously been prescribed. I told him that I'd have to talk about the situation with his mother.

Peter's mother and I had a conversation. It was obvious that homeopathy would have to wait a bit. First, we had to find a way to control Peter's multiple substance dependence. This would have to include some drastic measures like detoxification and rehabilitation. This was perfectly fine. First things must come first. Peter had to break his habit.

I saw Peter a few years after that. He found me on the Internet and came back, this time to my private office, sober and willing to receive treatment. The last time I checked, he was thriving.

Alcohol and Substance Abuse

Unfortunately, I've seen numerous cases when not only teens but also parents see nothing wrong with a sixteen-year-old getting drunk a few times a week or smoking pot. According to statistics from the National Institute of Alcohol Abuse and Alcoholism, 26 percent of eighth graders, 40 percent of tenth graders, and 51 percent of twelfth graders report having drunk alcohol within the past month. Sixteen percent of eighth graders, 25 percent of tenth graders, and 30 percent of twelfth graders reported binge drinking, which is defined as having five or more drinks in a row.

The Office of National Drug Control Policy (ONDCP) reports that according to the 2001 National Household Survey of Drug Abuse 10.8 percent of children ages twelve to seventeen are active drug users (a 9.7 percent jump since 2000). Among those who were heavy drinkers, 65.3 percent also used illicit drugs.

Certainly, the absolute priority is cleaning these children up, a process that always requires suppressive treatment of some kind. By the way, the theory of self-medication, which is popular with some addicts as a way of taking the responsibility off their own shoulders, in my experience, is true only in one way: people with underlying mental problems typically choose the wrong drug. People who feel depressed drink, even though alcohol makes them only more depressed. People prone to violence use PCP (also known as angel dust), which makes them more violent. Children with poor concentration who smoke marijuana get even more spacey and distracted.

If your child drinks or uses street drugs and doesn't want to stop, drug counseling and conventional medications are the way to go.

Quitting Cold Turkey

To be fair, I have to tell you another amazing story from my practice. Many years ago, I worked in a clinic where we had a few very sharp young ladies staffing the front desk. Johanna was a beautiful sixteen-year-old from Holland. Her life was well organized and under control. The only problem she'd ever had was with severe asthma. She used inhalers all the time and missed many days of work. I suggested trying homeopathy. She agreed. After an initial consultation, the remedy was very clear.

Then a miraculous cure occurred. Two nights after she took the dose, Johanna had a severe aggravation. Prepared by me, she used her inhaler. She didn't have to go to the emergency room. Things turned around after this initial aggravation. In a week, Johanna was able to stop using her inhaler all together. She was ecstatic because she was able to work out. Then, a month later, Johanna had a new attack. I invited her to my office to see what I could do. After about fifteen minutes of questioning, Johanna asked, "Dr. Shalts, could it get worse from pot?"

I answered, "Yes!"

It turned out that since a very young age Johanna had been smoking two or three *blunts* (marijuana cigars) a day. There is no detox for marijuana. Someone just has to stop. I informed Johanna of everything you've just read and gave her a repeated dose of her constitutional remedy. This time, she did OK for almost three months. It turned out that she was trying to quit marijuana. The quality of her life was improving daily.

After a third dose of the remedy, Johanna was able to stop. She's been doing well ever since. Interestingly, about a year later she brought her younger brother to my office. He was also a heavy marijuana smoker, who had developed severe depression after a death in the family. I prescribed the homeopathic remedy indicated for him at the time. A week later, this young man came back a picture of confusion. He'd stopped smoking marijuana cold turkey. I only had to give him a remedy indicated for his condition, and the issue was resolved. To the best of my knowledge, he is still doing very well.

Are these two cases exceptions from the rule? Not really. Both kids wanted to stop, and they did so with help from homeopathy. Nothing can make an addict stop, unless she or he decides to. As I said earlier, I've met families in which drinking and smoking pot are not considered wrong. For these children, the only way to go is conventional. We need to reserve suppressive treatment for suppressive, dangerous behavior. Sometimes we need to take a step back, so to speak, regroup, and then charge forward.

Admitting Your Child to a Psychiatric Hospital

One of our main considerations has to be the safety of a sick child. In some cases, hospitalization to the psychiatric ward is the only safe alternative. If the child is acutely suicidal or extremely agitated, just giving a medication—any medication, homeopathic or not—isn't going to resolve the issue. The child needs to be in a safe environment.

Parents, no matter how good their intentions, are not health care professionals. They don't know what to look for, or they simply might fall asleep when they should remain awake and watchful over a suicidal child. Parents also cannot restrain the agitated patient, even if it is their child. For serious situations, we need hospitals.

As I've mentioned a few times, the reality of life today is that conventional physicians provide all inpatient help. There are no homeopathic psychiatric hospitals in the United States at the present time. You should let the doctors do their job. Ignoring a serious, potentially life-threatening problem won't solve the issue. It will make it only worse.

After a dangerous episode is over and the child is discharged for outpatient follow-up, homeopathy can be introduced on top of conventional treatment and under the supervision of a psychiatrist. This is a safe way to go. The cavalier administration of homeopathic remedies to suicidal or agitated patients might result in an aggravation of the condition with initial worsening of the presenting symptom. Better safe than sorry!

Another situation when suppressive treatment in the initial phase is indicated is when the teenager doesn't want anything except conventional drugs. You should just make sure your child gets better. There are always later years of maturity when a person can make an informed decision about his or her own treatment.

When Suppression Is Wrong

Now let's talk about situations when suppression is wrong—very, very wrong.

First and foremost, there's absolutely no reason to medicate your child for normal variations of mood and sleep. I know it might sound silly to the majority of readers, but some members of the baby boomer generation have a tendency to medicate everything and everyone they possibly can. I've met very young children who were already on Prozac because parents "felt" that their child was "going through a difficult time," and some accommodating doctor went along with the idea.

I strongly recommend seeking homeopathic help first for treatment of ailments such as nightmares and night terrors, sleepwalking, various irrational fears, separation anxiety, and the initial uncomplicated stages of depression. Homeopathy does miracles in these areas. Of course, it would be highly desirable to work with a homeopath who is also a psychiatrist, but there are very few practitioners of this ilk. Another option is to connect your psychologist or psychiatrist with a homeopath and let them try to sort things out.

Homeopathic Treatment of Children Receiving Conventional Psychotropic Medications

Obviously, the ideal scenario would be to treat a medication-naive patient each and every time—that is, a child who has never taken any conventional drugs. In such cases, symptoms are crystal clear and no suppression is going on. It's easier to pick a remedy.

I am beginning to meet more children whose parents decide to bring them to me before a trial of conventional drugs begins. In some cases, I get more than a month to show results, which is a good trend in my practice. But the reality of the modern lifestyle is such that an overwhelming number of patients—over 80 percent in many homeopaths' estimation—including children, come to homeopaths after they've been prescribed conventional medications. Frequently, they're already taking more than one drug.

A number of homeopaths suggest discontinuing conventional medications first, waiting until the original picture of the illness the child has reemerges, and then administering a homeopathic remedy. Although absolutely correct and pure in theory, this approach seems to be unrealistic for the majority of cases. It's hard to imagine any parents who would risk the discontinuation of a conventional medication that helps their child even a little. Most of us realize that we have to be content with the present state of affairs and cope the best we can with our significantly more complicated cases.

The Cautious Approach

By suppressing or changing the original symptoms of an illness—or masking them all together—conventional medications can confuse the authentic *remedy-picture* of an illness. As we all know, the age of children who are put on strong medications, such as Ritalin and Prozac, is getting younger and younger. This issue is so serious that Roger Morrison, M.D., one of the leading American homeopaths, gave a special presentation on it at one of the annual conferences of the National Center for Homeopathy.

A number of homeopaths I respect use an approach that I believe is safe for handling the problem of blending homeopathic remedies with conventional drugs. Morrison named it the *cautious approach*. In this technique, a homeopath tries to find the best remedy while the patient is taking the conventional medication and then, as the child's target symptoms improve, gradually decreases the dose of the conventional drugs.

Tapering a child off a conventional medication doesn't necessarily have to be done by a homeopath. I'm sure that the conventional physician who prescribed the medication in the first place will be glad to see that the dosage can be decreased and perhaps totally eliminated sometime in the future.

In my experience, as the homeopathic remedy begins to work and a patient doesn't need a conventional drug anymore, more side effects or new side effects in many cases flag a need for the drug to be stopped. For instance, I've treated a number of teenagers with anxiety disorder. They came to my office on significant doses of anti-anxiety medications that have sleepiness as a potential side effect. As the homeopathic remedy I prescribed them began to do its work, these teenagers became lethargic and had to ask their doctors to cut down their doses of the conventional drugs.

Remaining on Conventional Medications Is Sometimes Wise

Some patients benefit from continuing conventional medication for an extended period of time. For example, sixteen-year-old Stanley came to my office after being treated by a conventional psychiatrist for a first episode of mania. His initial presentation was very intense and involved significant agitation and mania. He came to his initial appointment with me on four different medications: Valproic acid, a mood stabilizer; Risperidone, an antipsychotic; Benztropine, a medication that prevents side effects from Risperidone; and Bupropion, an antidepressant.

After six months of homeopathic treatment, all the medications except for Valproic acid were successfully tapered. Stanley, his parents, and I mutually decided to keep this one medication on board for a while. He couldn't promise complete sobriety while he was away at college, and he had a family history of bipolar disorder on one side and depression on the other side. Three years later, he's still doing very well. One day, we hope to be able to decrease and eventually discontinue the last drug. But we're in no rush. The main objective is to keep Stanley stable and free of mania and depression.

Seizing a Window of Opportunity

In some cases, the patient and the homeopath are offered a window of opportunity to use homeopathy without any conventional drugs. This used to happen frequently with Ritalin. Schoolchildren were given permission to take a break from the drug over their summer holiday, because they didn't have to be in school. Ritalin discontinuation usually doesn't cause physical withdrawal. Because that was the case, many children were able to do away with it.

The Art of Balancing Medications

I can compare the art of prescribing homeopathy on top of conventional medications with potato-sack racing. Jumping down a field in a burlap bag may be an interesting sport, but it requires skills different than simply running to the finish line. Anyway, most medically trained homeopaths seem to be getting better and better at it.

Naturally, most conventional drugs work in the opposite direction than homeopathy, as they suppress symptoms. That's why homeopaths will sometimes suggest that children on conventional medications take their homeopathic remedy more frequently than children would in "pure" cases—perhaps once a week or once a day instead of just once or once every few months. We need to constantly adjust the course of healing that periodically gets derailed.

Your homeopath will know how to handle such situations.

Attention Deficit–Hyperactivity Disorder

Attention deficit disorder (ADD) and attention deficit–hyperactivity disorder (ADHD) are terms intermittently used to describe children who have significant difficulties with concentration and effort. These children are impulsive and have trouble regulating their level of activity. They require frequent redirection and prompting.

The main credit for describing ADD goes to Canadian psychologist Virginia Douglas. She was one of a few scientists who studied the condition in the 1970s. As a result of her work, the names ADD and ADHD became mainstream in the 1980s. Since 1987, American psychiatrists have called the illness ADHD. Most recently, there's been an understanding that hyperactivity isn't necessarily present in all children with this illness. So now we distinguish three major categories:

1. ADHD, predominantly hyperactive type
2. ADHD, predominantly inattentive type
3. ADHD, combined type

Actually, the oldest recorded description of symptoms of ADHD dates all the way back to 1844. That year, Heinrich Hoffmann, M.D., wrote a poem in German entitled "The Story of Fidgety Phillip."

> *"Let me see if Philip can*
> *Be a little gentleman;*
> *Let me see if he is able*
> *To sit still for once at table."*
> *Thus spoke, in earnest tone,*
> *The father to his son;*
> *And the mother looked very grave*
> *To see Philip so misbehave.*
> *But Philip he did not mind*

His father who was so kind.
He wriggled
And giggled,
And then, I declare,
Swung backward and forward
And tilted his chair,
Just like any rocking horse;
"Philip! I am getting cross!"

See the naughty, restless child,
Growing still more rude and wild,
Till his chair falls over quite.
Philip screams with all his might,
Catches at the cloth, but then
That makes matters worse again.
Down upon the ground they fall,
Glasses, bread, knives, forks and all.
How Mama did fret and frown,
When she saw them tumbling down!
And Papa made such a face!
Philip is in sad disgrace.

Where is Philip? Where is he?
Fairly cover'd up, you see!
Cloth and all are lying on him;
He has pull'd down all upon him!
What a terrible to-do!
Dishes, glasses, snapt in two!
Here a knife, and there a fork!
Philip, this is naughty work.
Table all so bare, and ah!
Poor Papa and poor Mama
Look quite cross, and wonder how
They shall make their dinner now.

In 1902, British pediatrician George Frederic Still (an interesting name for a researcher of restless children!) reported the characteristics of children with aggressive, defiant behavior. They were hard to discipline and had difficulty paying attention and staying on task. Still suggested that the main reason for these behavioral problems was a birth injury. Despite this idea, the illness was labeled *morbid defect of moral control*.

After the 1917 to 1918 encephalitis pandemic, many children who recovered developed symptoms similar to those described by Hoffman and Still. This observation further strengthened speculation that this type of behavior is the result of brain damage. The illness was renamed *post-encephalitic disorder and minimal brain damage*.

As happens frequently with theories, it was shown that the children didn't have brain damage. So then, the name was changed to *minimal brain dysfunction*. Conventional medicine didn't offer any efficacious treatment for it until the 1950s, when there was a boom in the use of psychiatric medications. Stimulants were "rediscovered." By the mid-1960s, they were common medications for hyperactivity.

About that time, Stella Chase and some others hypothesized that *hyperactive child syndrome* was biological in nature. Even so, the American Psychiatric Association (APA) established a new diagnostic category: *hyperkinetic reaction of childhood*. Chase's colleagues largely disregarded her work, and the condition was believed to be the result of bad parenting.

During the last couple of decades, the fashion of applying a psychoanalytical label to all psychiatric illnesses faded away. Currently, the majority of scientists and physicians believe that ADHD is biological by nature.

Conventional Treatment for ADHD

The National Institute of Mental Health proposes that 3 to 5 percent of school-age American children have ADHD. It's absolutely the most commonly diagnosed disorder of childhood. The problem is diagnosed three times more often in boys than in girls.

One of the most disturbing occurrences of our times is that very often teachers, and even teachers' assistants, push parents to initiate treatment of their children with stimulants. Many patients of perfectly normal children hear, "Your son needs Ritalin."

Ridiculous! Prescribe stimulants just because a four-year-old has fun running around in preschool, or just because a healthy six-year-old runs around during recess? We really need to find a way to stop this disturbing practice.

If you think what your child's teacher says is correct, I strongly recommend that you take your child in for psychological testing. Measure twice; cut once. Medication should be the last step you take after plenty of appropriate evaluation. Teachers are not doctors.

Don't let family physicians or pediatricians just hand you a prescription. They aren't qualified to diagnose your child on this level. Giving out a prescription is easy, but what about all the consequences of labeling a child with any kind of illness? Or what about giving the wrong drug and not knowing what to do next? I can't even begin to tell you how many parents rush off to a local doctor or a neurologist to get stimulants. A psychiatrist or other doctor who specializes in ADHD must see your child.

Another alarming trend is the abuse of stimulants by teenagers who don't exhibit signs of ADHD. Any such drug has a high potential for abuse. For instance, a number of college students who routinely cram for exams take Adderall or Ritalin to help them stay up and think well. They do this in order to process large amounts of information in a short period of time. But after they take the test, their energy crashes—they sometimes even forget what they learned. And then they do it again. In the process, some get addicted.

We don't know what causes ADHD or the mechanism that cures it. Popular in the past, the theory of the *paradoxical effect of stimulants* has been abandoned. This theory referred to the calming effect on restless children caused by a stimulant (Ritalin), which is not unlike the principle of similars. Today the most popular theory connects ADHD with dopamine, a basic brain chemical.

Certainly, the mechanism of ADHD is complicated, and most probably new theories are going to emerge and disappear in the near future. There have been anecdotal reports of children cured of ADHD by taking allergens out of their diets and others demonstrating benefit with the addition of essential fatty acids like fish oil to the diet. Conventional biomedical research denies any connection with food or allergies.

Conventional medical books and medical journals report a very high (up to 70 percent) success rate in treatment of ADHD with Ritalin-like medications (stimulants). The National Institute of Mental Health conducted a study on the efficacy of these medications and reported satisfactory results in the treatment of attention problems and hyperactivity. However, a large proportion of children with ADHD also show symptoms of depression, anxiety, and sleeplessness. Ritalin and similar medications can make all of these types of symptoms worse. Even if Ritalin doesn't make them worse, it certainly doesn't make them better. That's when polypharmacy comes into play.

It is fairly common to have a child with ADHD on a few medications: a stimulant for attention and restlessness, an antidepressant, and a medication for sleep. If the child has an "anger issue," another medication, such as an antipsychotic, could be added to the list. Each of these medications offers a wide range of side effects.

These results might seem satisfactory to us, if we didn't know any better. Let's see what homeopathy can do for children with complicated cases of ADHD.

Constitutional Treatment for ADHD

We need to remember one important thing, the child—even if he is on his very best behavior and can concentrate very well—will get worse almost immediately after an allopathic medication is discontinued because conventional medicines don't cure anything—they only work while you take them. Homeopathic remedies provide long-lasting relief.

Frequently, there are issues, such as bed-wetting or nightmares, which come in the same "package" with ADHD. A homeopathic remedy frequently provides relief from these problems too, because it affects the health of the child on every level. One of the important benefits of homeopathy here is that it offers a child additional benefits for the same "price." The child takes just one homeopathic remedy for all his problems. This makes sense. After all, we treat the whole person, not just a particular symptom.

By contrast, the additional benefits of conventional medications are side effects. Some side effects are classified as desirable. For example, an antidepressant with sedating side effects might help with sleep. Remember, however, that it does not treat insomnia. It merely forces the child to sleep for the duration that he takes the drug. A few days after the drug is stopped, the insomnia comes back.

I met a boy named Eddie when he was ten. Most of his schoolmates and teachers considered him slow, and they all had their reasons. He was an unhappy, obese child who got teased a lot. He took a long time to answer his teachers' questions even when the rest of the students knew the answer right away. He also perspired constantly, especially on his forehead, which gave the impression that thinking required a huge effort. Although Eddie was a patient boy and tried not to show how painful his peers' remarks were, he was just a child and felt he must defend his pride. Fighting became a routine part of his daily activities. He would go to school, children would start teasing, and then he would stand up for himself physically. He didn't know another, better solution. The constant fighting provoked numerous complaints from children, their parents, and his teachers.

His family loved Eddie very much, but his home life was troubled. Eddie was afraid of being alone in the dark and had frequent nightmares, so he could only fall asleep in the same bed as his older sister. Although his fifteen-year-old sister loved him, sleeping in the same bed with Eddie wasn't a pleasant experience for her. Eddie still wet the bed, and his head perspired so much that the pillow was always damp and had a sour smell. Eddie also was very restless; he couldn't sit still when he was in class or at home doing homework. He also couldn't concentrate on most of the subjects he was being taught, except for the ones he really liked.

At the suggestion of his teachers, child psychiatrists had seen Eddie. They diagnosed him with ADHD and prescribed Ritalin for him and then other medications. But Eddie didn't get better. The situation at school got more serious. Eddie was becoming more isolative and angry. Because some of the medications he took caused unpleasant side effects, after a few trials his mother gave up. They were facing the possibility that Eddie would get suspended unless his behavior improved.

At this point, I heard the story from Eddie's mother. It came out in a casual conversation. I suggested trying homeopathy. I'd seen children with problems similar to Eddie's and knew that homeopathy often can provide a resolution to most, if not all, of them. After learning that the treatment was natural and couldn't hurt her son, Eddie's mother agreed to bring him to see me. She wasn't sure whether or not Eddie would agree. He was afraid of doctors, and he was very stubborn. But Eddie really liked his sister, and she was the one who convinced him to come.

One Saturday morning, I met with Eddie, his mother, and his sister, who came along, eager to help resolve the problem. She wanted freedom as much as Eddie's mother wanted him to get better. Eddie didn't seem to care. I thought he was depressed. A few things caught my attention right away. His T-shirt was soaking wet around the neck and at the waistline. Surprised by this phenomenon, I asked what was going on. Eddie showed me how he kept wiping his perspiring forehead with the midsection of the shirt. Another unusual thing was that most of this ten-year-old boy's front teeth still hadn't come in. After spending almost two hours with the family, I prescribed one dose of the remedy *Calcarea phosphorica* (calcium phosphate) in 200C potency.

Eddie was reluctant to take the pellet. But after he saw that the pellet was made from milk sugar, he agreed. I suggested meeting six weeks later to evaluate the progress of this treatment. Eddie's mother and sister were very skeptical. All I had done was listen to the story, watch Eddie carefully, and ask a lot of questions about his habits, such as what he liked and disliked to eat, how he slept, what his fears were, and such. To them, the process appeared superficial. In reality, I had to put an enormous amount of effort into identifying the remedy. It wasn't an "easy" case to crack.

Very often, a homeopath has to employ all the experience he or she has and all the knowledge that's available from other sources. An older homeopath once told me, "For me, the most challenging part of prescribing is to figure out what the patient doesn't say." That was true in Eddie's case. First of all, I didn't believe that Eddie really qualified as someone who needed to hit other people. His core problem was that he needed more time than others to process information and feelings. I factored in that he was stubborn and easily offended. But still the information I had wasn't enough to find the right remedy. There were too many potentially helpful remedies to choose from at this point.

Then the fact that Eddie perspired a lot on his head, that his perspiration smelled sour, that he was obese, and that his whole demeanor of being a stout, slow boy—even with teeth slow to come out—swayed me toward the *Calcarea* family of medications.

When I discussed this case later with another homeopath, she asked, "Why *Calcarea phosphorica?* Why not *Calcarea carbonica* (calcium carbonate)?" It was a very good question. Both homeopathic preparations are derivatives of calcium. Both share the characteristics of slow development (Eddie's front teeth still hadn't come in), introversion (Eddie had that), stubbornness (Eddie definitely had this characteristic), and many fears. (Eddie was afraid of the dark and of being alone.) But *Calcarea carbonica* is usually indicated for children who are anxious and cautious. Eddie was restless and had a capacity to fight back. Those last two characteristics are more strongly related to *Calcarea phosphorica.* It was a better match. That was why I made the choice that I did.

Can you see how very slight differences can weigh heavily in my decision-making process? Ultimately, I'm drawing on deep knowledge of the *Materia Medica* and my clinical experience to ferret out these subtle distinctions in my patients' symptoms.

Eddie's extreme fear of doctors and medications, his chronic unhappiness, and other people's perception that this boy had a bad attitude also directed me toward this particular preparation, *Calcarea phosphorica*. As in the case with Idis, in my head I had a virtual picture of both *Calcarea carbonica* and *Calcarea phosphorica*. The first was only a partial match. The second presented an ideal match.

Yet again, I feel I have to remind you that you are reading information digested by me after the fact. Analyzing this case was actually a difficult and laborious process. In the *Repertory*, the rubric (category) *concentration difficult*, which means "poor attention" in homeopathic language, lists three hundred remedies. And this rubric needed to be combined with at least two other rubrics: absentminded and daydreaming. Then this symptom had to be cross-referenced with all the information I presented previously in the chapter, which emerged through casual conversation, questions and answers, and purposeful observation.

From the moment you learned that this boy was cured with a single dose of a mineral, I am sure that you've been wondering, "How does it work?" You know what? That is a million-dollar question. We don't know the mechanism by which homeopathy works. Hahnemann was convinced that homeopathy works on a dynamic or—as we would call it today—an energetic level. The action of homeopathic remedies is so deep that it is obvious that they are affecting us holistically.

Homeopathy's systemic action cannot be explained by any hypothesis that involves a purely mechanical view of the body. Explanations that have been offered to date by biomedical science still have to do with "hardware" in our bodies, such as organs and cell receptors, whereas homeopathy probably has more to do with "software," aspects of our being that we presently can't appreciate.

In many ancient healing traditions, there's recognition of the life force called *chi* or *prana,* which is called Vital Force. Hahnemann adhered to this thinking, too. He strongly believed that this was the level on which homeopathy worked.

It is the fate of humanity to live with unknowns. Where does our million-dollar question leave us? We should strive to discover how things are, while continuing to use effective methods of treatment. Relentless research will reveal homeopathy's secrets.

Although homeopaths cannot offer a new, scientific-looking hypothesis of how remedies work, I can tell you that two hundred–plus years of clinical experience provide evidence that the constellation of symptoms similar to what Eddie was presenting to me respond well to a preparation of calcium phosphate. But if the substance weren't prepared homeopathically or administered according to the principle of similars, it wouldn't be curative.

As you can see, to find a remedy for Eddie, not only did I have to take a detailed history and collect as much data as I could through observation, but I also had to process all of this information by studying homeopathic tools, such as a computerized *Repertory* and the *Materia Medica*. Then, it is important to note, I had to apply my best clinical judgment and draw upon many years of past experience. What Eddie's family thought looked strange and kind of superficial was the result of two hours of hard work on my part.

In practice, the first remedy that's chosen for the child isn't always a perfect match. But this doesn't represent failure. It's a step in the constitutional healing process. Before a selection is made, the homeopath usually has a few remedies in mind. The practitioner must be sensitive to ever-so-slight differences between similar homeopathic remedies. In some cases, the first remedy removes a layer of problems that the homeopath observed during an interview, thereby uncovering a whole new perspective on the child that more closely matches a different remedy. The child now presents a clearer picture. This guides the practitioner to ask more questions and place greater emphasis on different symptoms. In a follow-up visit, the homeopath reconsiders and chooses from among the other potential matches. More than one meeting may be required for a homeopath to observe, as well as ferret out, the details that lead to prescribing the simillimum. The next case we'll discuss explores exactly this type of process.

Two weeks later, I met Eddie's mother in the street by chance. She was happy to see me. She told me that five days after taking the remedy, Eddie took all of his stuff out of his sister's room and went to sleep in his own bed! She was amazed. I asked her to wait and see how long the change would last.

Six weeks later, Eddie and his family came for a follow-up appointment. Eddie looked happier. He obviously felt much better about himself. He could sleep in his own bed. His bed-wetting issue had improved. His head perspired significantly less. Most of his front teeth were coming in! More important, he could do his homework faster and he was participating in the class. His teachers and his classmates were surprised at how different Eddie had become. Life was beautiful!

Needless to say, Eddie's sister was also very happy. Eddie and his mother wanted more of the medication. To their surprise, I suggested waiting. From my perspective, there was no reason to give more, as the remedy was working. Eddie was capable of taking care of his health on his own. He was free of illness and free of medication.

Eddie came for a few more follow-ups at intervals of a month or two. At some point, the family went thorough a significant crisis and Eddie felt worse. He told his mother that he needed to see me. The remedy he needed remained the same. I simply repeated the dose and Eddie got better in a few short days. This happened years ago, and I don't know where Eddie is now. One thing is certain: homeopathy changed his life.

I know that this story might sound fantastic to you. As I've remarked, miraculous cures like this one keep homeopaths enthusiastic about what they do. Many situations are significantly more complicated than Eddie's and require longer treatment. But it's clear that homeopathy offers a cure, so a child doesn't need to be on strong drugs all the time.

As you've probably noticed by now, I try not to give out the names of remedies that I use for the treatment of a particular illness. In this chapter, I made an exception, mainly because Eddie's case is so spectacular, and the remedy prescribed wasn't a simple choice to make. Please don't get stuck on the particular remedy I gave to Eddie. Many remedies can be used for the treatment of ADHD or any other illness.

The choice of the remedy, as I'm sure you know by now, depends on the individual characteristics of the person who is being treated. A typical mistake is to try to figure out the remedy based on symptoms common to the diagnosis. In allopathic medicine, this approach is the rule. In homeopathic medicine, this approach leads us to select the wrong remedy.

Persistence Pays Off

I would like to emphasize the fact that homeopaths have to have enough time to find a cure. It isn't always easy. And even if the first remedy chosen works just fine in the beginning, a second prescription of a different remedy might be necessary to advance the healing process even further. Here's another example from my practice.

Stan was an intense eight-year-old. Teachers, students, and even his parents had to walk on eggshells around him, as he was extremely explosive. He would hit or even bite at the smallest provocation—or sometimes without any provocation. But this was only one side of him. Another side was that he was afraid of many seemingly benign things, like the dark and dogs, for example.

Stan would never go to sleep with the lights off. Frequently, he woke up screaming with an expression of horror on his face. Going to school was a big task for Stan. He couldn't concentrate or sit still for a long time. As happens relatively often, this severe presentation of the illness presented a very clear picture of a remedy to me.

I gave Stan a dose of *Stramonium* 200C (which is made from the thorn apple, a warm-climate plant that varies in size from herbs to shrubs, and even trees). This remedy is indicated for children with a constellation of symptoms that includes severe nightmares, fear of the dark, and fear of dogs, as well as the tendency to overreact in a violent way. Of course, many other smaller details about Stan fit into the puzzle that formed a clear picture of this remedy in my mind. Five days later, his concerned mother phoned me to say that Stan was completely unable to sleep and he was very scared. I explained that it was a healing crisis, and no matter how cruel it might seem, we just needed to wait it out for a few days. Three nights later, the aggravation subsided. Stan started sleeping better, and his behavior at home and at school improved.

At the follow-up appointment six weeks later, Stan's mother was very pleased to report that Stan's teachers were happy about the progress he was making. There was no hitting or biting. We decided to wait.

At the next follow-up appointment, I heard from his parents that Stan was becoming clingy. He wanted to be hugged a lot. They also told me that his food habits, body temperature, and the position in which he slept had changed. Now Stan wanted creamy, sweet food. He asked for butter and ice cream every day. He started sleeping on his back and became so warm that he kept kicking the covers off. Those changes would have been fine, except for the fact that he was also experiencing eczema similar to a case he'd had when he was two years old. His parents had forgotten to mention that to me.

As we discussed earlier in the chapter, all the new information clearly indicated that Stan now needed to receive another remedy. This time, it was *Pulsatilla nigricans* (also known as the wind flower, a thick, woody, acrid-tasting plant native to the dry soils of Northern and Central Europe). Fortunately, most people don't settle in the state of *Stramonium*, as it's scary. After initial treatment, children usually get better and frequently require a different remedy to complete their constitutional cure. Stan went from a state of terror and the need to attack, to a state of being soft and needing company and comfort. Combined with the changes in his appetite, sleep position, and body temperature, these symptoms created a new mosaic that clearly translated in my mind into the clinical picture of *Pulsatilla*. One dose of *Pulsatilla* 200C gradually brought about the resolution of the issues just described. Since then, Stan has been doing great in general, with occasional colds that respond beautifully to homeopathic treatment when indicated.

Of course, there's an element of trial and error involved in the process of homeopathic prescribing. But homeopaths know what we need to do to narrow the odds in the patient's favor. We know how to approach people, how to research remedies, and how to determine what symptoms to look for. We do the best we can, holding in mind that our objective isn't just to throw a medication in someone's direction and hope it produces a cure.

When I prescribe, I am not using an antidepressant medication *only* because a person is depressed. I am not using a laxative medication *only* because a person is constipated. I am looking for a simillimum for the person, not for the illness. My goal is to find a remedy that will treat depression or constipation in a particular person, after taking all of that person's individual characteristics into consideration. This is called *differential therapeutics*. It means I'm never using a remedy blindly. The choice is never random.

There are certainly some cases when the remedy that solves the puzzle of the case is not obvious right away. An experienced homeopath will be able to play a game of homeopathic chess to figure out the remedy that will result in restored, natural good health.

Anxiety

Conventional psychiatry distinguishes a group of emotional problems called *anxiety disorders*, which includes generalized anxiety disorder, separation anxiety disorder, phobias, panic disorder, obsessive-compulsive disorder, and post-traumatic stress disorder. We should remember, especially in the case of teenagers, that illegal drugs and drug withdrawal also cause severe anxiety sometimes. In addition, certain physical illnesses, such as hyperthyroidism, can cause symptoms of anxiety.

Generalized Anxiety Disorder

Children and adolescents with generalized anxiety disorder suffer from extreme, unrealistic worries about everyday life activities. They become like old babushkas. They worry unduly about their grades, the health of their relatives, and about being late for school. Many young people with this problem complain of feeling tense. They also frequently complain about stomach problems or discomfort in other parts of their body. Physical exams and tests often come back negative.

Separation Anxiety Disorder

Children who suffer from separation anxiety have difficulty leaving their parents to go to school or a camp. Often they cling to their parents and don't want to stay home alone. They can only sleep with their parents, even when they're six years of age or older.

Phobias

Some children have unrealistic and excessive fear of certain situations or objects. Many such phobias have been given specific names, depending on what the specific fear is. Many children are afraid of animals, thunderstorms, water, heights, or narrow spaces like elevators. Children and adolescents with social phobia are terrified of being criticized or judged harshly by others.

Panic Disorder

Panic attacks are periods of intense fear accompanied by a pounding heartbeat, sweating, dizziness, nausea, or a feeling of imminent death. Repeated panic attacks in children and adolescents without a cause are signs of a panic disorder.

Obsessive-Compulsive Disorder

OCD is characterized by a pattern of repetitive thoughts and behaviors. OCD sufferers are aware of how bizarre the thoughts or actions are, but they cannot stop them. Compulsive behaviors may include repeated hand washing; counting; or arranging and rearranging toys, DVDs, or other objects.

Post-Traumatic Stress Disorder

PTSD is becoming more commonplace nowadays. It results from surviving scary, traumatic experiences. The events of 9-11, living through a hurricane or an airplane crash, witnessing a friend or relative killed, or being the victim of physical or sexual abuse are examples of such experiences. Children who suffer from PTSD experience the event over and over through strong memories, flashbacks, and nightmares. Their emotions are usually extreme. They also often worry about dying at a young age.

Conventional Treatment for Anxiety

Anxiety disorders are common in children and adolescents. About thirteen of every hundred children and adolescents age nine to seventeen have some kind of anxiety disorder. Girls are affected more than boys. Separation anxiety disorder is reported to be present in one out of every twenty-five children. OCD is present in one out of every two hundred children.

As you can easily see, even from the little information provided here, some children present only a few relatively mild problems, whereas others are very ill and need all the help they can get. If your child is scared of large dogs but everything else is OK, most probably no treatment is indicated. However, if the fear affects your child's life, making normal functioning close to impossible—for instance, your child has to stay home all the time—treatment needs to be prompt.

As with any other kind of emotional problem, medication isn't the only solution you should be seeking. Psychological intervention is also important, and the sooner the better. An experienced psychiatrist will be able to guide you through the initial steps of treatment, which should include a workup to exclude the possibility that illicit drugs or a physical illness are causing the problem. This step is very important. If a teenager is on drugs, the use of any treatment modality is bound to fail until the teen cleans up.

The conventional medications used to treat these conditions in children are exactly the same medications that are used to treat adults. The main type prescribed to achieve long-term results is antidepressants. Drawbacks are that these medications take weeks to produce a significant effect. They have numerous side effects. They also must be taken for many years or even a lifetime.

For immediate, temporary relief from anxiety, children can be offered benzodiazepines, such as Clonazepam, Lorazepam, and Diazepam. These drugs can be highly efficacious for anxiety, but they are sedating and highly addictive.

Homeopathic Solutions

Homeopathy offers an excellent alternative to conventional drugs. Obviously, a clear benefit is that homeopathic treatment doesn't require a child to stay on a remedy forever. Before I talk about examples, I would like to point out that there are exceedingly normal children and adults who share a tendency to worry more than other people. As long as this habit doesn't affect daily life, no treatment is indicated.

Let's see what homeopathy has to offer our children.

Jordan came to my office by accident. I met his father at a mutual friend's party. After learning that I am a board-certified psychiatrist, he asked me whether I could do anything to help his thirteen-year-old son, and he gave me the following details.

Jordan seemed to be constantly preoccupied and constantly worried. When asked what was going on, he would answer that he had the same thought going through his head. He also had to repeat certain activities every day. Before leaving for school, for example, he had to touch the door exactly five times in the exact same spot, and then he had to walk five steps forward and five steps backward. He also had to repeat certain words many times in a row before he felt that he could sit down at the dinner table. Pretty disorganized before the problem arose, Jordan absolutely had to have certain things on his desk in a certain order now. He was also very anxious and couldn't concentrate at school. All of these problems had started cropping up about a month after the attack on 9-11. Jordan had seen the footage on TV and had gotten very upset.

I explained to Jordan's father that I practice homeopathy and I'd be glad to help, but he needed to understand what I do clearly. I recommended a book to read. Soon after our conversation, he set an appointment.

When Jordan and his parents came to my office, I could tell that Jordan was a quiet, timid young man. He told me that something weird was sitting inside of him and "this thing" controlled what he was doing. He couldn't stop thinking about this problem. He was tormented by it, preoccupied with these thoughts all day and night. He felt depressed and had developed vertigo, which was much worse in the morning. He also felt dull. Often he caught himself forgetting why he'd gone to the kitchen or what he was looking for in a drawer. His concentration was terrible. Formerly happy, easygoing, and sharp, now he was constantly afraid that something bad was going to happen to him or to his family. He wanted to stay around people all the time.

The family was seriously considering heavy-duty psychiatric medications. The conventional diagnosis of this condition would be PTSD with strong elements of OCD. Preoccupation with this "thing" that was telling Jordan what to do also could have been classified as a delusion—maybe he was hallucinating. The selection of conventional medications could have been daunting and likely would have included an antipsychotic.

I was fortunate to identify the right remedy for Jordan. He needed *Mancinella*, a rarely prescribed remedy that's derived from the *Hippomane mancinella* (Manzanillo, a euphorbiaceous tree that grows from Mexico and the West Indies through Colombia). Provers of the herb reported feeling that something inside "took over" them, as if they were "possessed." That was how Jordan told me he felt. It is a well-established fact that many different plants can alter perception and cause hallucinations. The effects of LSD, marijuana, and some mushrooms are common knowledge. *Mancinella* doesn't have any abuse potential. Still, the majority of provers reported this strange and unusual symptom, which is why a remedy made from this plant would be appropriate for someone like Jordan. I knew that children sometimes go into this kind of delusional state after watching horror movies or experiencing real-life horror. And I was correct. The *Mancinella* worked beautifully for him. Jordan's symptoms gradually went away. In two to three months, he developed a new picture of a different remedy, which finished up his healing process. He has been doing very well ever since.

Finding such a remedy requires detailed knowledge of homeopathic medications and an extremely clear understanding of what's going on inside the mind of the patient. It seems highly improbable that someone—a parent, a patient, a layperson—could identify a need for this remedy simply by collecting a bunch of facts and plugging them into a computer. Generally, people look for what they know; and this was unusual.

Because I practice in New York City, I've seen a number of children with PTSD that developed after 9-11. Homeopathy literally does miracles for such cases. It's a pity that so few people know about homeopathy and that even fewer appreciate how helpful it can be.

Shyness and Separation Anxiety

Of course, not all cases of anxiety disorders are so grim. I also see children with mild separation anxiety, stage fright, and panic attacks. Homeopathy helps tremendously.

Why don't we talk about Lana, a sweet little girl I saw when she was seven? Lana had a few different problems. She *really* wanted to stay with her mother all the time. And she was generally very shy, especially with strangers. When she came to my office, Lana spent one hour, two-thirds of the appointment period, sitting on her mother's lap. She was kind of coquettish, as she blushed a lot. Her mother told me how Lana's life was limited because of her shyness and separation anxiety. We spoke about Lana, I observed how she was, and then, at the end, Lana felt well enough to say a few words.

The remedy was pretty clear. After a single dose of the remedy in a concentration 200C, Lana started to become more confident. By the end of the first month, she was able to go to school without much of a problem. Our follow-up appointment was easy. I didn't see any new symptoms and decided to wait. In the course of a year, we only had to repeat the remedy once, when Lana had a cold. Today she's doing just great!

Panic Attacks

In Part Two, you learned about a few possible remedies for acute fears and anxiety. Some of the same remedies can help many chronic cases, too. A few years ago, I saw a young gentleman named Andy in my office. He was ten at the time. He'd felt scared most of his life. In fact, when I met him in the waiting room, he seemed to be so scared and shaken by the entire experience that he couldn't sit still. He had an expression of sheer terror on his face. I knew I had to give him something to help him calm down. In my opinion, Andy had a clear case requiring *Aconitum napellus*.

Interestingly, anyone who had read Part Two and learned about *Aconitum* would probably have been able to identify Andy's acute need for this remedy. Earlier in the book, we spoke about how acute prescribing can often spare parents and children a lot of grief. "A stitch in time saves nine." One of the most basic, well-known remedies, *Aconitum* is frequently needed in cases of severe panic. It would have saved Andy trouble if it had been given immediately after an initial event that scared him profoundly.

The main characteristic of people who need this homeopathic remedy, and of provers and victims of monkshood poisoning, is severe, uncontrollable fear accompanied by restlessness. Andy fit this description perfectly. It indicated to me that he'd respond quickly to the remedy. *Like* cures *like*, remember?

If *Aconitum* were the simillimum for Andy's symptoms, his mind and his body—his whole being from the core to the periphery—would respond to it positively. I wish I could tell you why, but no one knows for sure. To date, science hasn't been able to reveal the mechanics of homeopathy. However, research studies reported in prominent peer-reviewed medical journals, including the *Lancet* and the *British Medical Journal*, have demonstrated homeopathy's clinical effectiveness.

But was there such an event in Andy's life? I was hoping to find out after my patient calmed down. Who knew, maybe he needed a totally different remedy to resolve his chronic problem. I gave him *Aconitum* in potency 200C. Then I invited Andy and his mother into my office, where I gave Andy some toys.

His mother told me that similar episodes happened very frequently. The worst thing for Andy was riding an elevator. The subway was absolutely out of the question. Airplane flights had never even been considered, as his parents knew that Andy wouldn't be able to tolerate them. The trouble had started when the boy was four. While playing on the street, he was suddenly approached by a large dog. Although the animal only wanted to play, it scared Andy. He was literally terrified—and stayed in that state of terror for years. Various treatment approaches, including antidepressants, had utterly failed.

I've actually seen a few similar cases in adults, such as a young woman whose severe panic attacks started after a garden tool chopped off a part of her foot when she was six years old. In her case, to calm her down, I also had to give *Aconitum*.

By the end of my assessment, Andy was feeling more comfortable. I was also very comfortable. In my assessment, the boy had already received the right constitutional remedy. He needed *Aconitum*. The positive effect of that remedy persisted for a long time. Obviously, *Aconitum* is only one of a few hundred remedies that may be indicated for various people with anxiety and panic disorder.

There is no doubt in my mind that homeopathy offers very effective treatment for various types of anxiety disorders.

Autism

A famous book, *Wild Boy of Aveyron*, by Harlan Lane, tells the true story of an unusual boy, captured by peasants near the village of Lacaune, France, in 1797. He was dirty and couldn't speak. He moved like an animal, on four extremities. The locals put him up for public display, but he escaped. Recaptured in 1798, he was taken to the home of a widowed woman in the village, where he was clothed and fed for a week but escaped again at the first chance. The boy became known as Victor. In 1800, when he showed up for food during a harsh winter, he was again captured. Eventually, he was taken to Paris and examined by renowned psychologist Philippe Pinel, who denied that the boy could have been brought up by beasts. Pinel pronounced Victor an incurable idiot.

A young physician, Jean-Marc Gaspard Itard, who worked with deaf and retarded children, took Victor under his care. With his help, Victor learned to read, to say a few words, and to obey a few simple commands. He never learned how to speak properly. This boy has become a symbol of the first case of autism known to medical science.

Leo Kanner, M.D., published the first official scientific description of autism in 1943. Prior to Kanner's work, such children were classified as emotionally disturbed or mentally retarded. Hans Asperger, M.D., identified a different group of children, who had characteristics similar to the ones described by Kanner, with the distinction that they had the ability to speak. The term *Asperger's Syndrome* now describes autistic children with speech. Kanner borrowed the word *autism* from a famous psychiatrist, Eugene Bleuler, who also coined the term *schizophrenia*.

How to Recognize Autism

Autism is a complex developmental disability, characterized by defects in ability or an inability to interact with other people, defective or even absent communication skills, and a restricted repertoire of activities and interests. Many people who work with autistic children feel that they are very intelligent. The main problem, at least for other people, is that the autistic child doesn't communicate with them in the way most people do. Sometimes they don't communicate at all. A large proportion of autistic children also have significant behavioral problems, frequently with elements of aggression.

You should become concerned if your child exhibits these characteristics:

- Does not babble or coo by twelve months of age
- Does not gesture (point, wave, grasp) by twelve months
- Does not say single words by sixteen months
- Does not say two-word phrases without prompting by twenty-four months
- Has loss of any language or social skill at any age

Many resources are available to parents of autistic children, including so-called early-intervention programs and autistic centers, which are rapidly growing in numbers.

The number of cases of autism is rapidly growing in the United States and around the world, although it is unclear whether the actual number or merely the rate of diagnosis has changed. Many people call it an epidemic. Let's take a look at some statistics. There was an 805 percent cumulative growth rate in the diagnosis of autism from 1992 to 2003, with a 20 percent average annual growth rate for the same period. One out of 264 children was diagnosed with autism in 2003.[1]

Some studies indicate that not all children with autism are included in statistics. One study reported that only 50 percent of children with *autistic spectrum disorders* had autism listed as their special learning designation. Parents are extremely concerned about the increasing incidence of this very serious disorder. Autistic spectrum disorders are disorders that have many symptoms in common, including autism, Asperger's syndrome, Rett's disorder, and childhood disintegrative disorder, among others.

Many theories of the origin of autism have been suggested. Some people blame vaccinations, mercury, food allergies, infections, brain defects, and so on. The truth is that we simply don't know what is causing the apparent rise in this terrible illness. People are just recycling the usual suspects. From the homeopathic point of view, a particular subpopulation of children has a predisposition to respond to a number of stressors, including a few just named, with a particular constellation of symptoms.

I've rarely seen cases of autistic children where a particular incident was the definite trigger of a severe reversal of already developed communication skills. The majority of my patients with autism had no obvious trigger. I've seen many families that had more than one autistic child. Frequently in such a family, only the first child receives vaccinations. With the second child, the parents don't give the vaccination because they think there might be a link. But the second child is still autistic. Autistic children are all different and present with different combinations of various typical features as well as simply normal variations of individual characteristics that all other children have.

Some practitioners have been offering parents homeopathically prepared vaccines to be used for "detoxification" from the negative effects of conventional vaccines. Because there is no hard proof that there is a definite link between vaccination and autism, and because there is no proof that these protocols are efficacious, I don't recommend them. They may even harm children. This process isn't classical homeopathy for two reasons. First, it is not individualized. Second, it is polypharmacy.

Conventional Treatment for Autism

Let's talk first about the conventional treatment of autism. Occupational, physical, and speech therapies are extremely helpful and should be integrated, if possible, in the treatment schedule of every autistic child. Behavioral and educational treatment modalities are also important.

The list of psychiatric drugs given to these children, some very young, looks pretty scary. It includes antipsychotics, antidepressants, stimulants commonly used to treat ADHD, and mood stabilizers commonly used to treat bipolar disorder. All of these medications are used as a single or a multiple prescription to suppress various symptoms that autistic children have. This treatment is not based on any theory whatsoever. The goal is "to improve quality of life."

Of course, some children become quiet and less restless when taking these drugs, but none of these medications touches the core of the problem. None affects their ability to interact better or to speak. I'll quote C. T. Gordon III, M.D., a professor of psychiatry at the University of Maryland Medical School. His article was published in *Advocate*, November-December 2000, a publication for parents of autistic children: "There are no medications that directly address cognitive impairments such as language difficulties or deficits in abstract thinking and social understanding. . . ." Research in this area continues. It is well funded and I hope it has, as Gordon concludes, "a very bright future."[2]

Many parents who are disappointed in conventional treatment seek alternatives. These methods include megadoses of various vitamins, Secretin injections, hyperbaric oxygenation, and such. David Nathanson is considered to be the first one to have tried dolphin therapy in the 1970s. Many parents report significant changes in their children after the contact with dolphins. As with many other illnesses, no single method has provided consistent results in autistic children.

Homeopathic Solutions

In my experience, which is limited to a few dozen patients, the most efficacious combination is homeopathy and cranial therapy, with the additions of sensory integration techniques, occupational therapy, and behavioral therapy. Children also significantly benefit from going to specialized schools.

One of the prominent audiologists in New York, Dr. Jane Madell, tells the parents of the children that she refers to me: "Go to Shalts. He gives children *Tarentula*. It's weird, but it works." Obviously, I don't give everyone with autism a homeopathic preparation of *Tarentula*! I only give it to those who have symptoms that indicate the need for it.

Remedies that help autistic children don't have to be exotic—not at all. I've had cases that responded to such remedies as *Sulphur* (sulphur), *Belladonna*, and *Pulsatilla*, and I've used some preparations from the animal kingdom. I select these remedies pretty much the way I make my selections for children with any other illnesses.

Recently, I treated a four-year-old boy named Daniel, who had absolutely no language abilities and didn't communicate with his parents at all. A few doses of *Sulphur*, a basic homeopathic remedy, brought about an amazing change in him.

Of course, children with autistic disorder uniformly strike people as severely ill and disconnected. On some Web sites, I've read that the main remedy for these kids is *Helleborus* (the early blooming shade perennial more commonly known as the Lenten Rose), a statement that's the result of a superficial understanding of homeopathy. One of the words used to describe the symptoms that this remedy cures is *stupefaction*. If people plug that or other common signs of autism into a computer search program, *Helleborus* will be one of the frequent selections.

As you know by now, a homeopath has to look for qualities that make a person different from everyone else with the same diagnosis. Daniel struck me as someone who was happy and easy-going. He had a good appetite but hated fish. He was thirsty for cold drinks. He would ask for food every day at 11 A.M. He really hated bathing. This little boy also had stools so offensive that they smelled up the entire house. Daniel's parents told me that he'd had a fairly severe diaper rash on his little behind as a baby. It was bright red and itchy. Every now and then, he still had a tendency to develop slight eczema. Daniel was very warm all the time. He would kick off his covers at night and refused to wear many layers of clothing. All these pieces of data, which are totally useless to a conventional physician and seemingly unimportant to a layperson, gave me a pretty clear picture of the remedy Daniel needed.

Obviously, lots of children hate fish, many are thirsty, and many don't like to bathe. But a constellation of all these symptoms is a different story. The fact that Daniel once had diaper rash in a particular location and that it was so angry confirmed my prescription. I went looking for whatever made this boy different from everyone else who doesn't speak, and I found it. And that's why I gave him *Sulphur*, which is made from the element sulphur (not the antibiotic sulfa). I made a choice of this particular remedy because every single unique symptom that Daniel had corresponded to its characteristic symptoms. They came together tightly to form the picture described by many provers of *Sulphur*. Although there's no single homeopathic remedy for autism, there was no reason to look for anything more exotic.

Why did the *Sulphur* work? How come such a simple mineral preparation helped an autistic child to become more connected and develop language so quickly? I hate to sound like a broken record, but the truth is that we don't yet know the mechanism by which homeopathic remedies work. One thing is clear: the mechanism of healing—the principle of similars—is universal. But individuals need different remedies to stimulate their healing processes. The remedies we give to different autistic children vary because we know that different children respond to different energetic signals.

In two months, Daniel developed eye contact and started making sounds. Four months after that, he developed a vocabulary of sixty words. Another three months later, he had over three hundred words in his vocabulary and was using two-word phrases. At the next three-month follow-up appointment, Daniel had an almost normal conversation with me and even placed all the toys he'd been using back in the basket at the end of our interview.

I was fortunate to study with Paul Herscu, N.D., who has probably seen more autistic children than anyone else in the United States. He introduced us to the idea of the possibility of treating this population of people. There are presently a number of homeopaths that treat autistic children with success. Finding a remedy for these children is very difficult. Frequently, their communication with the outside world is minimal. One needs to be able to see ever-so-slight individual characteristics of these children to find a remedy that is specific for this very special child. I have to say that I see some improvement in every autistic child whose parents follow up on a regular basis. Some children get better to a spectacular degree. Others slowly improve and finally come to the point when they can communicate their needs and even develop language skills. Their behavior gets progressively better. I've also seen failures, when I couldn't achieve any visible results. Please understand, I always assign the failures to my limitations as a practitioner. In cases like that I always keep on trying to find the correct remedy. Homeopathy has been shown again and again to be very efficacious. But in some cases, finding the correct remedy, the magic simillimum, can be very difficult.

I decided not to present many clinical examples in this chapter, as I don't want to give details about a few miraculous cures, which may mislead you and raise expectations.

Homeopathy definitely works for autistic children. In most of the cases, it's a difficult process, in which a child gradually improves, becomes more attentive, has no aggression, and gradually develops communication skills. I currently have a patient, a little three-year-old girl, who cannot speak at all, and who illustrates this process.

When she came to my office six months ago, her motor skills and even her gait were very poor. She also was totally disconnected from other people, including her mother. She definitely has significant neurological defects and barely fits a definition of so-called autistic spectrum. In a sense, her problems are much worse than that. After a few doses of one remedy, this little lady has been able to improve her motor skills. She started to learn and then mastered sign language.

The last time I saw her, we played ball for only a few minutes. For the little girl and her parents, this was huge progress. Is she going to speak? I don't know. Is she getting much better? Absolutely!

As with other cases, periodically I meet parents who expect instantaneous results. "We have a month before we start Risperidone, and we decided to try homeopathy."

This is an impossible challenge for an autistic child to handle and very difficult for a homeopath to accomplish. If you decide to give homeopathy a chance, please give your homeopath at least as much time as you gave some inefficient care provider that you met beforehand! Of course, you may lose the battle with autism again, but you (and especially your child) may also win big.

Depression

According to a fact sheet for physicians posted online by the National Institute of Mental Health, depression now occurs in children at an earlier age than in past decades. Recent studies indicate that early-onset depression continues into adulthood. More than that, childhood depression increases the chances of having significant health problems in adult life. Depression in children is also associated with an increased risk of suicide.

In a bizarre twist, we recently learned that antidepressant drugs—the same conventional medications being used to treat depression—increase the risk of suicide in children. The FDA issued a public health advisory about this topic in October 2004.[3] This advisory was based on studies of nine antidepressants, including

SSRIs, in children and adolescents with major depressive disorder (MDD), obsessive-compulsive disorder, or other psychiatric disorders. They also mandated that the manufacturers of these drugs add boxed warnings to labels and package inserts.

Signs of Depression

The picture of depression in children can be quite different from the adult picture. Some depressed children pretend they're sick so they don't have to go to school, or they express a worry that their parents may die. Their grades often decrease significantly. Teenagers may start getting in trouble at school and become grouchy and negativistic, or they feel misunderstood. Sometimes you may hear, "Your child changed," from a teacher. Teenagers may get involved in promiscuous sexual activity and alcohol and drug abuse.

By the way, the situation with drugs and alcohol works in reverse, too. Children who use drugs and alcohol often become increasingly depressed.

In our day and age, drugs have to come to your mind first in every case of sudden, unexplainable changes in your child's mood and behavior. I've seen amazing cases when even hospitalized teenagers were able to fake a urine test checking for the presence of drugs, but their mood and behavior changed dramatically without any treatment because they were sober.

The main symptoms of depression are the following:

- The child is feeling sad or is crying a lot without any relief.
- There are feelings of guilt for no reason, a loss of confidence.
- Life seems meaningless or it's as though nothing good is ever going to happen again. A child develops a negative attitude or behaves as if she has no feelings.
- There is a loss of interest in things that the child used to like, such as music, sports, being with friends, and going out. The child wants to be left alone most of the time.

- The child becomes forgetful and has difficulties with concentration.
- There is a marked irritability. The child flies off the handle with minimal provocation.
- The child is either very sleepy, or there's a loss of sleep.
- Appetite is either increased or decreased.
- The child talks about death or dying.

It also isn't uncommon to develop bipolar disorder (manic-depression), in which episodes of severe depression alternate with periods of feeling so great that someone has no need for sleep and tons of energy. Mania is always followed by an emotional crash.

If you suspect that your child is depressed or manic, you need to act fast. At any suspicion of suicidality, call 9-1-1 and stay with your child until help arrives. Treatment of depression has to be conducted by highly trained professionals.

Please heed this *warning: suicidal patients must be hospitalized.*

The best combination is for a child to receive psychotherapy and a homeopathic remedy or a conventional drug if homeopathy isn't an option. Unfortunately, I've even heard five- and six-year-olds talk about dying.

Homeopathic Solutions

The homeopathic treatment of depression is quite effective. I've treated a large number of teenagers and children with depression with consistently good results. This includes the many cases when my new patients were already on conventional medications.

Usually, children on medication come to me because they either have shown no improvement or because they experienced severe side effects. The rule of thumb is to continue the antidepressant, start the homeopathic remedy, and then as the child gets better, gradually taper off the conventional medication.

It's not uncommon in my practice to wind up seeing an entire family in which a sibling and both parents suffer from depression or bipolar disorder in addition to my patient. Remedies don't need to be repeated frequently for depression, even in patients who are on conventional medication already. As always in homeopathy, the key is to identify the right constitutional remedy.

His parents brought John to my office when he was fourteen. It was an emergency visit. A few months earlier, he had started mentioning that he wanted to die. Things at school were bad. The family had just moved to a new house in a town far from where they'd lived before. John had really been looking forward to the move, as the new school was supposed to be much better. But the loss of all his old friends affected him deeply. Then he wasn't able to make new friends because he became withdrawn.

Reserved by nature, John became very quiet and didn't initiate contact with anyone. When at home, he spent most of the time in his room. His parents knew that he slept very little. His appetite decreased. John complained to me that when he lay in bed all night, he kept thinking the same thought over and over again.

After learning that he wanted to die, his parents took John to the hospital. Following a relatively brief hospitalization, he was discharged on an antidepressant. Fortunately, there was no suicidality anymore. But John developed numerous side effects. His sleep became even worse, so he was prescribed a sleeping pill by an outpatient psychiatrist. Now, on top of everything else, he was sedated.

The choice of the remedy was actually pretty clear to me. John received one dose of *Natrum muriaticum* in concentration 200C. As you can see, John received the same remedy that Idis did, discussed earlier in the chapter. He also had many features characteristic of *Natrum muriaticum*. The presentation may seem different, but on a deeper level the issues are still the same: problems with separation, constantly looking back, being withdrawn, feeling isolated, and depression. If you remember the analogy with Lot's wife, it still applies here. God told her not to look back and she did anyhow. People who need *Natrum muriaticum* have this tendency to dwell on the past.

So *Natrum muriaticum* is the remedy for depression, right? After all, it worked for both Idis and John, didn't it? Not necessarily.

There are 547 remedies that potentially can be helpful to people with depression. *Natrum muriaticum* is one of 53 that are indicated more often than others. Still, the choice was made on a combination of different symptoms that had to closely match the entire picture of the proving of *Natrum muriaticum*. It was only after that happened that I made my final choice.

This case clearly illustrates the point I've made before. A homeopath that has experience in prescribing the same remedy to different people often can easily identify its picture. But without experience and a good knowledge of homeopathic remedies, the search for a remedy may become an endless, fruitless venture.

After our work together, I referred him to an excellent psychologist who works well with children. John had instructions to check in with me every time he didn't feel well. Reserved patients actually prefer e-mail communication. In rare cases, I allow this type of communication. It's certainly better than nothing! He sent me e-mail.

Gradually, John got better. I never needed to change the remedy. But at the follow-up appointment four weeks after his first visit, I repeated the dose of the original remedy once because his symptoms of depression started coming back.

At the next four-week appointment, we began tapering him off the sleeping pill. By the time John came back the next time, he was sleeping a bit better, and we started bringing down the level of the antidepressant drug. We did this over the course of a few months. It has been four years now. John is doing fine.

What else can I say? Homeopathy works!

In the last chapter, we'll explore treating chronic physical problems with homeopathy.

Chapter Nine

Treating Chronic Physical Problems

In this final chapter of the book, we'll explore the topic of constitutional treatment for chronic physical problems, including allergies, earaches, sinusitis, asthma, eczema, and obesity. As you know, homeopathy is powerful medicine that treats various illnesses at a deep, core level by stimulating a healing response in the body.

What Can Homeopathy Do for Severe Chronic Physical Problems?

When talking about the treatment of physical problems, it's especially important to remember that the body heals itself naturally. With the exception of surgical procedures and the use of mechanical devices, such as reading glasses, hearing devices, artificial limbs, and artificial organs, medicine is supposed to provide a better environment to support this innate capacity.

Homeopathy does a great job in creating a supportive healing environment. When expeditiously treated with homeopathy, an acute condition goes away without leaving any ground for a chronic problem to flourish. Allopathic drugs, in contrast, not only suppress acute symptoms—often without completely eliminating their underlying cause—but also cause side effects, which, in essence, present a new, different illness.

Antibiotics are supposed to kill or weaken bacteria, and they usually succeed. But our own defense mechanisms do the true "dirty work." Our bodies finish the process of eliminating the intruders, clean up, and then—most important—restore normal functioning to the diseased organ. Unfortunately, in the case of antibiotic treatment, our immune system might also need to deal with the side effects of antibiotics, such as allergic reactions. One problem gets fixed, and another problem gets initiated. The majority of people put up with this, because they think there is no other choice: "There is always a price to pay." But the susceptibility to illness is unchanged, and the next batch of bacteria may be resistant to the antibiotic.

The Importance of Treating the Whole Person

The human body has an enormous, fantastic capacity for self-restoration and regeneration. A naive belief that the body is similar to a machine that could simply be mended on a mechanical level is plainly wrong. But even in a device, such as a car, which is relatively primitive when compared with any sophisticated biological system, a malfunction of one part will cause reciprocal malfunctioning of many other parts.

Consideration of the interconnectedness of the parts of complicated systems is critical in the development of medical treatment strategies. Obviously (at least to me or any other holistic practitioner), concentrating all the attention on one particular organ and ignoring the rest of the body is a mistake and cannot yield good results.

Pardon me for the analogy, but putting new tires on a car without realigning its four wheels may seem to be enough to fix the immediate problem—the car can go—but in the long run this may cause new problems; elements of the power train could go bad and result in even larger distress for the owner. I'll never forget how a poorly fixed radiator in one of my favorite cars essentially ruined the engine. The price asked by a mechanic to fix the new problems that arose forced me to get rid of the car.

A half-done job on a human body causes significantly more problems, and the problems tend to crop up significantly faster than they do in machines. More important, we cannot exchange our bodies. We'll never have another one—not in this lifetime. So we must be exceedingly careful and considerate of the bodies we do have.

Here's an example from conventional medical practice that illustrates this point. When I was in the ninth grade, I had a friend named Max. He was an interesting guy, both very smart and very good in sports. One day, he fell during a soccer game. No big deal. In a few minutes, he felt OK and continued to play. But a few hours later, he developed a severe pain in his right arm. It was so severe that his concerned father took him to the pediatric outpatient clinic. The pediatrician examined Max and—without ordering an X ray—said that there were no "typical" signs of fracture. According to him, all that Max needed was some rest and painkillers. "Most probably," the doctor said, "it's muscular pain."

A few days went by. Max still couldn't use his arm, and his father took him to a specialized orthopedic clinic. After examination by an orthopedic surgeon, the picture was clear. Max had a fracture. But the treatment was significantly more complicated than it would have been if he'd arrived sooner, because Max's bones hadn't been repositioned right away. The process he endured then was painful, and the healing was long.

This is a clear example of what can happen if a doctor doesn't know what to do. The interesting thing is that even excellent conventional physicians sometimes don't know what to do. Orthopedic surgery is the rare example of a situation in which everything about a condition is generally clear: fracture, treatment, success, and no negative consequences. In the majority of other medical cases, nothing is clear. The exact mechanism of illness often is unknown.

Why Does Disease Occur? Two Points of View

Although there may be numerous hypotheses about reasons for disease and mechanisms, the body is so complex that nobody knows exactly what's going on in the body most of the time. Even in the case of infectious diseases, some people get sick and some don't. Why? Why do some children get asthma, or sinusitis, or skin diseases? We don't really know.

Conventional medicine proclaims that suppression of all its symptoms cures a disease. We've spoken about this before. We also discussed the consequences of suppression: rather than being cured—eliminated from the body—an illness grows deeper roots and becomes chronic.

Who's to say that eczema and asthma are disconnected? Let's go along, for a moment, with a theory that conventional medicine offers and accept that both of these illnesses are the result of allergies, a defective immune response. If so, the eczema is a response on a superficial level and the asthma a response on a deeper level. It wouldn't be a good idea to convert a child with eczema to an asthmatic.

Unfortunately, the problem doesn't stop at this level. Frequently, significant emotional issues accompany a chronic illness that's considered physical, such as asthma or a food allergy. You and I know why. It's Hering's Law. The direction of cure has been suppressed—and possibly reversed—by conventional treatments. This is how a relatively superficial illness moves into the level of the deep vital organs and ultimately to the core of the human being: the mind and emotions. This is not a very comforting state of affairs!

Conventional medicine offers drugs that at their best cause remission. This means the temporary improvement of a chronic illness. The price tag for this outcome, which is the best you can get with conventional treatment, is having a child who constantly needs to take drugs. Medications cause side effects that often have to be treated with other medications. The vicious cycle continues. Predictably, a suppressed physical illness will crop up on the emotional level. It's plain to see. Unresolved physical problems always change people's moods, energy levels, and general outlook in life. A homeopath appreciates all these issues.

Homeopathy doesn't provide an answer to the ultimate question: Why does disease occur? It's an unfortunate reality, but nobody knows a single root cause for sinusitis, asthma, or any other chronic ailment. Yet homeopathy has an approach that allows us to tap into the mystery of an illness. By perceiving the patterns of imbalance in the sick person's body, we find a remedy that leads to complete healing. A homeopath is concerned with providing assistance that will lead to elimination of the core issue, not just to suppression of symptoms. Homeopathy celebrates the wisdom of nature. Allopathic medicine forces a hypothetical view of disease on patients, causing permanent dependence on medication and ultimately the worsening of overall health. Homeopathy offers patients independence from drugs and disease. The majority of chronic childhood diseases respond well to homeopathic treatment.

By utilizing homeopathy for acute conditions, we can prevent children from developing chronic conditions in the first place. Those who are already suffering from chronic illnesses can be cured with homeopathy. "Cured" means becoming disease-free, enjoying restoration of normal functions of the body without needing medications.

Allergies

As I was writing the book, a friend told me that her five-year-old niece isn't allowed to bring a lunch to her school that contains dairy or nuts. And it's not because she has allergies to these foods. It's because other children with allergies might get sick if this little girl shares her lunch with them. Doesn't this sound insane to you? How many children suffer from the problem of food allergies?

An Increasing Phenomenon

Allergies are the sixth leading cause of chronic disease in the United States, costing the health care system $18 billion annually. More than fifty million Americans suffer from allergic diseases. Eight percent of children younger than six are intolerant to different foods.

Allergic dermatitis, an itchy rash, is the most common skin condition in children younger than eleven. Scientists report different estimates. Between 9 and 30 percent of the population are suffering from this illness. Hives are also common. Ten to 20 percent of the population have them at some time in their lives. Half of those affected continue to have symptoms for more than six months at a stretch.

Allergic reactions account for 5 to 10 percent of all adverse reactions to drugs. Penicillin is a common allergen, or reactive agent. Approximately 7 percent of healthy volunteers develop a positive allergic reaction to penicillin in skin tests. Although the true number of deaths from drug reactions is unknown, anaphylactic reactions to penicillin occur in thirty-two of every one hundred thousand exposed patients.[1] Think about it. Now we are taking for granted that our children, as a result of treatment that is supposed to relieve their acute conditions, can frequently develop a different, chronic illness. This is reality in twenty-first-century America, or any other developed country.

The Assault on Our Children

Fifty years ago, allergies were rare; only a few children had hay fever or other allergic reactions. Today teachers keep anti-allergy medications in their classrooms.

There are a few explanations for this phenomenon. On the one hand, our children's immune systems are assaulted on a daily basis by various chemicals that have polluted the environment for years. On the other hand, the uncontrolled and unnecessary use of antibiotics is a major contributing factor in the development of hypersensitivity. A number of people also point to excessive vaccination as a probable cause.

We need to remember that children in the so-called civilized world have little or no contact with unpolluted nature. Figuratively speaking, their immune systems don't have experience with the process by which the bodies of children throughout history were able to figure out what is a friend and what is a foe.

The field of immunology has made significant progress in understanding how these things work. In short, our immune system has two armies of lymphocytes. B-lymphocytes react to outside intruders. They are the body's CIA. This is the part of the immune system that is most affected by environmental pollution.

T-lymphocytes monitor the internal situation. We can call them the immune system's FBI. They are largely responsible for the elimination of defective cells and other biological substances that are produced by the body itself.

Obviously, if the agents of these two systems, the lymphocytes, never had experiences with foreigners, they might mistake our own healthy cells and friendly substances, like milk, eggs, and wheat, for enemies—and develop a reaction to them. The term *sensitization* is used to explain how substances like antibiotics can predispose the lymphocytes to overreacting to other, frequently normal substances.

When they weren't at school, children in the 1950s and 1960s played on the street most of the day. Their hands were not so clean, and they constantly touched dogs and cats. Their immune systems very quickly learned to recognize what was a friend and didn't overreact to these substances. Their exposure to environmental pollution, antibiotics, vaccination, and such was minimal or nonexistent. People now in their mid-forties and younger weren't sensitized to normal environmental factors. Breast-feeding ensured that friendly bacteria would inhabit a child's gut. Healthy bacteria, such as lactobacillus and acidophilus, provide training that's important to the immune system.

Today you can still find this healthier lifestyle in some developing nations. Sadly, allergies are one of the big prices we had to pay for our technological advances.

Scientists have found an interesting solution to this problem. They recommend introducing acidophilus bacteria very early in a baby's life. These bacteria do two good things. They compete (and win) against the bad bacteria that occupy the gut of bottle-fed babies. They also share characteristics of bacteria that children of the 1950s and the 1960s would normally have met on the street. This exposure trains the B- and T-lymphocytes to be more tolerant to what is good and to develop a stronger response to what is bad. This technique is a great idea and it yields good results, but it doesn't solve the overall problem.

Another interesting technique is called *desensitization*. This method is based on finding out what a child is allergic to and then giving the child the same substance in tiny doses. Doesn't it seem similar to homeopathy? This technique also has given some good results, but ultimately, because the individual characteristics of a child aren't considered in the process, the results are not as good as homeopathy.

The Homeopathic Solution

I hate to sound like a broken record, but homeopaths pioneered both the research and the treatment of allergies. In 1871, British homeopath C. H. Blackely suggested that seasonal sneezing and nasal discharge were the result of exposure to pollen. American homeopath Grant L. Selfridge, M.D., was the first president of the American Association for the Study of Allergy, which, after merging with the Association for the Study of Asthma and Allied Conditions, became the American Academy of Allergy. That organization was the predecessor of the present-day American Academy of Allergy, Asthma, and Immunology.

Homeopathy treats allergies with great success. We've developed treatment approaches to both acute seasonal and chronic allergies of many types. James Tyler Kent made a very important step in this direction. In a famous series of lectures presented at Hering College in Chicago, Illinois, he clearly defined the theoretical and practical principles of treating allergies. Usually, acute allergic reactions that people develop during the allergy season are treated first, and then, during the symptom-free season, a homeopath finds a constitutional remedy that solves the problem.

You might be surprised to learn how many cases of severe allergic reactions to bee stings have been treated with simple homeopathic remedies, such as *Apis* (honeybee). You know how to use this remedy (see Chapter Six) and you should do it, if such a situation arises.

I've encountered a number of cases when parents ask if I can help a child who is on antibiotics at the time and having allergic reactions to it. This scenario doesn't call for homeopathy. Homeopathic treatment cannot override damage done by an allopathic medication while the medication is still on board, so to speak. However, there are other steps, including the use of probiotics (that is, friendly microbes), which you can take. The time to see a homeopath is after the child's antibiotic treatment is over. Homeopathy has tools that help restore an immune system that's been damaged by antibiotics or short-term hormonal treatment.

Some children are born with numerous allergic reactions. Treatment of these babies is complicated, but my colleagues and I have seen excellent results. In some cases, one dose of a constitutional remedy does the entire job. In other cases, treatment takes significantly longer.

Frequently, children with allergies develop other local diseases, such as chronic asthma and sinusitis, which are considered to be mostly allergic in nature. Although it's nice to be able to permit your child to play with dogs and cats, some children are so allergic to pets that they cannot even be in a house if a pet was there earlier in the day. Homeopathy helps with that kind of problem.

An interesting article was published in the *British Medical Journal* in 2000.[2] A group of scientists from the Glasgow Royal Infirmary, a famous British homeopathic hospital, and from the University of Sydney in Australia, conducted a multicenter, double-blind, and placebo-controlled study of fifty patients. The study clearly shows benefits of homeopathic treatment when compared with a placebo.

In the same article, researchers reported the results of the statistical analysis of four independent studies pulled together—the current one plus three previous similar studies. The total number of patients was 253. This analysis also revealed a definite improvement after homeopathy, as compared with a placebo.

Another study, published in the *Lancet* in 1986, clearly demonstrated that a combination homeopathic remedy used for the temporary relief of allergic symptoms was significantly superior to placebo.[3] That study was conducted on only twelve patients, so achieving statistical significance is difficult.

Obstacles to Cure

A major obstacle in treating children with allergies is a parent's desire to try different healing approaches simultaneously. Some are fine. Some interfere with homeopathic treatment. Certainly, setting dietary limitations and removing the substances that trigger allergies is always a good idea at the beginning. But using hormones or other conventional allergy medications isn't helpful to the child who is starting homeopathic treatment. In some cases, the discontinuation of allopathic medications that the child is already taking can only be done gradually and at the same time as the administration of homeopathic medications. The process can be time-consuming.

Here is a description of one of the many cases of allergies that I've treated.

Theo was a very skinny and quiet six-year-old. He played peacefully with toys in my office while his mother told me his story. At a very young age, when he was only one, Theo developed an ear infection. It was treated with antibiotics. Then he had another one. Antibiotics again. I am not going to list every single case for which he was treated with drugs. Just take my word for it; there were plenty. I'm sure it's a common scenario. Gradually, Theo developed many allergic reactions. He absolutely couldn't be around cats. Although he liked animals, his parents were afraid even to have a dog; Theo might be allergic to it. He also had multiple food allergies. Basic foods like bread and milk were absolutely out of the question. Theo also had severe seasonal allergies. Sound familiar?

When I evaluated Theo, one of the striking features was that he was very quiet and serious. I asked his mother how Theo was before he developed allergies. She said, "He's been quiet since I can remember." Even his language skills hadn't developed before age two and a half. Interestingly, before he spoke English, Theo communicated through his own private language. Finally, Theo agreed to switch to English.

Many details of Theo's presentation pointed to *Natrum muriaticum*, a homeopathic remedy that helped this young gentleman overcome his physical problems. In Chapter Eight, you read two stories about children with emotional problems who required the same remedy. So wasn't it specific for depression? No. Then is it a specific remedy for allergies? Absolutely not! Although it is a tempting notion to believe a remedy could be a specific cure for an aliment, in fact this remedy—like the others—is only indicated for some people. It is right for those with allergies, depression, or migraine headaches, and other conditions that also exhibit the other symptoms it possesses.

You may think the way I phrase my comments about remedies is weird. "This makes no sense. *Natrum muriaticum* is just a diluted mineral. It has no feelings. It is not alive. Therefore how can it possibly *have* symptoms?" Homeopaths make such statements, because for us each remedy is associated with a virtual picture, meaning a picture in our mind's eye, that is a mosaic composed of symptoms experienced by various provers in original research experiments, and by patients who've been cured with *Natrum muriaticum* during the past two hundred years. We have a long history of successes.

The composite picture of the remedy is very lifelike. In a homeopath's mind, it has a life of its own. Its symptoms are represented throughout all the organs and all the systems of the body, because all biologically active substances affect the entire body, not only one organ. Everything is connected. In provings, volunteers reported symptoms on every level of their being—mental, emotional, and physical. Symptoms that can be helped with this remedy are exhibited on all the different levels of a human being.

If you think about the reality of allopathic medicine, the situation is exactly the same. For example, Valproic acid, which was originally used for the treatment of seizures, also helps people with mania. Medications from the group of beta-blockers, originally used for the treatment of hypertension, also help people overcome stage fright and anxiety. Thorazine, the first antipsychotic medication, also helps treat nausea and can decrease blood pressure. Side effects of the majority of conventional medications are represented in all major systems of our body and mind. Just read an insert from the package of any conventional medication and you'll see this for yourself.

Only homeopaths are able to take advantage of this phenomenon to treat the whole person, rather than just a single symptom. Let's take a few concrete examples from the homeopathic computer program called Radar. In the *Repertory* that's the basis of this program, symptoms are divided into forty-two different sections representing different areas of bodily function. *Natrum muriaticum* is present in all of them. Actually, *Natrum muriaticum* can cure numerous symptoms in each of the systems of our body. It has 1,054 symptoms listed in the section called Mind; 856 in the section called Head: 196 for the nose, 198 for the ears, 372 for the back, 90 for dreams; and 1,161 symptoms in Generals. As you may recall from reading earlier chapters of this book, mental and general symptoms are very important in choosing the right remedy.

Remedies are prescribed for the person with the illness, not for the illness. Different people, depending on their circumstances and stages of life, the kind of stressors they face, and the particular sensitivities and weaknesses of their bodies, may exhibit different sets of symptoms that are associated with the same remedy. That's what happens during provings, and that's the reality in life. Although books and Web sites may offer reader-friendly descriptions of various psychological states that apply to different remedies, this information is only partially accurate. It may be misleading to those who have no experience in homeopathy. Obviously, an experienced homeopath would be aware of all the different manifestations that a particular person may have.

I paid attention to Theo's symptoms and clearly distinguished a need for *Natrum muriaticum*, because he had so many of its characteristics. Yes, he had ear infections and allergies, as many other children do; he was also reserved, quiet, developed his language abilities late, and even had invented a private language first. In addition, the type of discharges from his nose and his food preferences played important roles in the selection of the remedy.

After a dose of *Natrum muriaticum* 200C, Theo lit up quite a bit. Six months later, most of his problems were gone. He also successfully handled the pollen that used to cause allergies in the spring. He didn't need any medications.

As time goes by, Theo is still becoming stronger. I hear from his parents on the rare occasions when he develops a cold. Homeopathy continues to help this little boy stay allergy-free.

Of course, *Natrum muriaticum* is only one of many remedies that might help resolve allergies. It wouldn't cure every child's allergies.

Eczema

Eczema is the most superficial of all serious chronic conditions. I'm not going to say that it's not a big deal. It is. If left untreated, a chronic illness of any kind can only go one way: deeper. Perhaps you have read that eczema in infants usually goes away by age two and a half. This statement is accurate. The trouble is that nobody ever knows where the eczema went. Did it just disappear, never to come back? Or did it hide, to come back a few years later in a different form?

Allopathic dermatologists clearly distinguish two main types of skin problems:

- Conditions related to diseases of the internal organs. Leukemia, tuberculosis, and Crohn's disease, for example, are often accompanied by a skin illness called *erythema nodosum*.
- Conditions that are considered to be purely skin problems, such as eczema.

Interestingly, most dermatologists strongly suggest that eczema has a clear-cut allergic component. So who's to say that a case of "disappeared eczema" means that there's no problem anymore? And who's to say that asthma appearing a few years after the disappearance of eczema isn't a manifestation of the same underlying issue?

Is it possible that after this symptom (eczema) goes away, another group of symptoms caused by the same imbalance in the immune system will appear on a different level? There are no prospective studies on that. No one knows the state of health of children who had eczema as infants. Maybe an even more important question is what happens to children who had suppressive treatment for eczema early in their lives?

Signs of Eczema

There is a broad term for skin inflammation: *dermatitis*. Eczema is a form of dermatitis. *Eczema* comes from Greek, meaning "to boil over." This description fits the picture of the illness pretty well. Eczema is an itchy inflammation of the skin that can be red, blistering, oozing, scaly, brownish, or thickened. Eczema is also frequently called *atopic dermatitis*, which means "allergic." Very frequently, this type of eczema is inherited and accompanied by hay fever or asthma.

As you can see, this single observation proves the point brought up earlier: the disappearance of skin symptoms doesn't mean that the deep-seated, underlying problem went away. There is also a term *contact dermatitis* or *contact eczema*. This type of skin disease is the result of a direct contact with a substance that irritates the skin. For instance, a very common form of acute contact dermatitis is poison ivy.

Eczema is artificially classified in smaller subgroups according to what seems to be the main cause of the illness. Obviously, such a classification cannot be too helpful. How come some people develop the illness and some don't when exposed to the same irritating substance, even an allergen or a chemical?

Different sources agree that in the last thirty years there has been a significant increase in eczema in children. Some say this is a twofold increase; others say fivefold. Sources offer different information on how large a population of children is affected. Some say eczema affects one in eight children (12.5 percent). Some say up to 20 percent.

Conventional Treatment of Eczema

As we all know too well, the main medications used for the treatment of eczema are antibiotics, antihistamines, and corticosteroids. The main objective of allopathic treatment is to control symptoms. Apparently, control is different from cure. It's also important to remember that conventional medications can cause complications that in some cases are worse than the original symptoms of the illness. As discussed earlier, antibiotics may cause a change in the population of friendly microbes that occupy the gut. These are needed both for normal digestion and the development of the immune system.

Corticosteroid hormones cause many problems. In my view, the worst one is mood changes. What would be better: Having clear skin and a depressed mood, or having a good mood and eczema? Can you even answer this question? Recently, the FDA approved the use of *nonsteroidal* medications, such as Pimecrolimus and Tacrolimus, to treat eczema. These drugs are approved for use in children two years and older. Although I'm not a dermatologist and have never prescribed these drugs, the list of potential complications seems pretty serious to me and includes some systemic conditions.

Without a doubt, there are cases of mild eczema that resolve spontaneously, and there are very severe cases that respond beautifully to conventional treatment, with all the symptoms of eczema being completely suppressed. What happens later on with the child's health remains to be seen.

Here's a warning: if your child develops significant inflammation of the skin, you should immediately contact your physician or dermatologist.

The safety of your child comes as an absolute priority. As I've said many times before, we don't have homeopathic hospitals or full-time pediatric homeopathic clinics in America right now. So at this time, all emergency issues have to be resolved promptly by going to see a conventional physician.

Homeopathic Treatment of Eczema

The paradox in treating this seemingly superficial condition with homeopathy is that it's difficult to treat, but perseverance brings about amazing results—a total cure. No more eczema and no asthma or any other systemic condition.

Many failures seem to be the result of parents' impatience with the progress of homeopathic treatment. They rush to blend other treatments into the mix and counteract healing. A big issue is that most children come for homeopathic consultation after they've been through a series of unsuccessful trials of allopathic medications. They also receive suppressive ointments. Parents have real trouble letting go of conventional methods, especially if they've perceived a degree of improvement (suppression).

If your child has eczema or any other skin condition, my advice to you is to try to start working on the issue with homeopathic treatment.

There are many homeopathic remedies that help cure eczema. But you should not attempt to select remedies for eczema on your own. Only a well-trained homeopath will be able to guide you and your child through all the steps of the treatment. Homeopathic combination remedies may be able to suppress some of the symptoms, but an ultimate cure can be achieved only by constitutional homeopathic treatment.

Untreated or allopathically treated eczema is frequently the first stepping-stone on the road to asthma. Along with chronic sinusitis, it's considered to be a significant predisposing factor to asthma. It also frequently accompanies asthma in very young children.

Sinusitis

Sinusitis is a huge health problem in both the pediatric and adult populations. According to current statistics, chronic sinusitis is the most commonly reported disease. The CDC receives reports of thirty-three million cases of sinusitis annually. Americans spend millions of dollars in search of relief for their disturbing symptoms.

Allopathic physicians divide sinusitis into three groups:

- Acute, which lasts for three weeks or less
- Chronic, which usually lasts for three to eight weeks but can continue for months or even years
- Recurrent, which means several acute attacks within a year

As you've probably guessed by now, the two last groups actually represent chronic sinusitis. It is interesting to note that even with all the treatment that's being offered currently by conventional medicine, sinusitis may last "up to a year."

Signs of Sinusitis

Sinusitis is an inflammation of one of the four pairs of cavities located in the bones of the skull that surround the nose.

- The *frontal sinuses* are located over the eyes in the brow area.
- The *maxillary sinuses* are located inside each cheekbone.
- The *ethmoid sinuses* are positioned behind the bridge of the nose and between the eyes.
- The *sphenoid sinuses* are located behind the ethmoid sinuses in the upper region of the nose and behind the eyes.

Allowing for the free exchange of air and mucus, each sinus has an opening into the nose. Each is joined with the nasal passages by a continuous mucus membrane lining. So anything that causes a swelling in the nose, such as an infection, an allergic reaction, or an immune reaction, also can affect the sinuses.

The mechanical part of the process that leads to the development of symptoms is well understood. As a result of an infection that leads to the swelling of the lining of the sinuses, air, pus, and other secretions get trapped within a blocked sinus and cause pressure on the sinus wall. That, in turn, leads to a sensation of pressure and pain. In another common scenario, when air is prevented from entering a sinus by a swollen membrane at the opening, a vacuum can be created inside the sinus that causes pain.

The Limitations of Conventional Treatment

Allopathic physicians understand perfectly well that several sinus cavities may be affected. They know that the location of the affected sinus dictates the symptoms that are present and where the location of the pain is. For example, an infection in the maxillary sinuses can cause aching pain in the upper jaw and teeth. Because the ethmoid sinuses are near the tear ducts in the inside corners of the eyes, inflammation of these cavities often causes swelling around the eyes and pain between the eyes. The sphenoid sinuses are less frequently affected. But if an infection sets in there, a child may complain of earaches, neck pain, and deep aching at the top of the head.

All this sophisticated information, which would help a homeopath understand a patient's need for a particular individualized remedy, goes down the drain when it comes to conventional treatment. The treatment arsenal of allopathic physicians doesn't allow for an individualized approach to curing either acute or chronic sinusitis. Instead their first line of attack is to combine a powerful antibiotic with a decongestant and a painkiller. Three drugs are regularly involved in the treatment of an acute episode.

Without a doubt, in cases of a first episode of acute sinusitis in a very healthy child with Level One health, or upper Level Two health, there's a strong possibility that the antibiotic will help eliminate the episode with no return of symptoms later.

Because children's sinuses aren't fully developed until age twenty, and their ability to localize pain and discomfort is not as developed as it is for adults, most children with sinusitis have pain or tenderness in several locations, and their symptoms usually don't clearly indicate which of the sinus cavities is inflamed.

In addition, the drainage of mucus from the sinuses down the back of the throat (postnasal drip) can cause further complications, such as throat infections. It doesn't matter. Allopathic treatment remains the same.

This situation clearly illustrates the limited ability of allopathic medicine to use the database of information that it has created. In contrast, homeopathic practitioners purposefully look for the differences between children with sinusitis. We know these differences are the very things that allow us to choose a specific remedy for a particular child with sinusitis.

Another important point is that the current theory of chronic sinusitis places the emphasis on the allergic component. In some materials, the connection between sinusitis and asthma is clearly established, with sinusitis preceding asthma. However, this doesn't change much in the medical approach to this debilitating, commonplace illness.

Self-help books offer many different ideas about prevention and how to manage sinusitis without medications. Some promise you a cure in the main title, but the subtitle clearly indicates that the book is talking about *relief* of symptoms, which is a politically correct way to talk about temporary suppression. Other books are more honest and talk about surviving the condition, which at least presumes that no unrealistic promises are being handed out. Authors of these books may give important and helpful advice on how to diminish the impact of this persistent illness. But they don't provide steps to a cure.

The Homeopathic Solution

Here's something totally "unrealistic." Homeopathy promises a cure for most cases of sinusitis, a real one. I am able to make this bold statement, because I am myself an example of such a cure. Mine came years after childhood ended. But for many children who have seen homeopaths, the cure is already a reality of life. I could tell you many stories about these children. All would look the same.

Essentially, the story is as follows. A child had an episode of acute sinusitis. The child took many antibiotics. Finally, the child had chronic sinusitis. The child was offered surgery. Then the child's parents decided to seek homeopathic help as a last resort. One dose of a homeopathic remedy made the child feel much worse in the beginning and then better and better, until no symptoms were present anymore.

In some cases, as you may have already imagined, the story is a bit longer because a few homeopathic prescriptions were required before the condition's ultimate resolution happened, a cure. There will always be a percentage of cases where a homeopath isn't able to identify a constitutional remedy for a particular child.

As a rule, cured patients don't come back to see the homeopath, so I cannot offer you a longitudinal case study on many of my own patients. Instead I've decided to tell you my own story. It illustrates the whole process of going through multiple experiences with conventional medicine.

I developed sinusitis at age four. My parents and I went for a summer vacation on the Black Sea. By the end of that trip, I felt weak and was sensitive to riding on the bus. It easily made me carsick. After going home, I developed a fever and a headache and was quickly diagnosed with sinusitis. Antibiotics were prescribed a few times with limited success. From then on, chronic sinusitis affected the quality of my life.

Throughout childhood, I had frequent headaches. As a complication of my frequent use of antibiotics and other conventional medications, I quickly turned from a very skinny child to a pretty heavy one. In the fifth grade, I had to undergo surgical drainage of my sinuses. Although local anesthesia was provided, this was an extremely painful procedure. About six months later, I had a set of similar procedures done as an outpatient. I had a talented eye, nose, and throat doctor, who did them well. He told me that at the rate I was going, I'd probably wind up needing surgery to put tubes in my nose. I continued to have sinus infections two or three times a year but never had surgery.

When I grew up, I practiced yoga rigorously for many years. I learned how to flush out my nose with saltwater, did headstands and breathing exercises, and was a vegetarian. The sinusitis seemed to have gone away. But after the stress of immigration to the United States and the discontinuation of my yoga practice, my sinusitis returned.

My first truly enduring break from sinusitis came after I was pre-scribed a homeopathic remedy by another homeopath in 1990. It went away until 2001, when it briefly came back, at which point another remedy was prescribed by a homeopath, and I have been disease-free ever since. How's that for long-term results?

My advice to you is definitively to see a homeopath for the treatment of your child's chronic sinusitis. But if your child is in the middle of a severe infection—a very uncomfortable condition—use antibiotics one more time. Make sure that your child is well and safe and then reach out for homeopathic help.

Asthma

Asthma has a profoundly disabling impact on too many children. It affects more than 4.8 million children in the United States, mak-ing it the most common serious and chronic childhood disease. Here are some facts:

- Asthma accounts for ten million absences from school each year.
- Asthma is the third most common cause of childhood hospi-talizations under the age of fifteen.

- More than two hundred thousand children with asthma experience more severe symptoms due to exposure to secondhand smoke.

- About ten million visits annually to office-based physicians result in a diagnosis of asthma.

- Asthma cases and asthma deaths have been on the rise. From 1979 to 1996, asthma deaths have risen 120 percent, from 2,598 to 5,667.

- Hospitalizations for asthma have increased 256 percent from 1979 to 1996, to 474,100 people annually.

- Asthma treatment costs an estimated $11.3 billion, including direct and indirect expenditures each year.[4]

How to Recognize Asthma

The most common way to find out that your child has asthma is to witness an asthma attack. The picture is terrifying for the child and for the parents. It can be described in a very simple way: the child cannot breathe.

Physicians know the mechanical aspects of the problem well enough. The membranes in the bronchi, the small branches of the main airways in the lung, become swollen, and circular muscles in the airways contract. More mucus is produced in the airways, and this makes breathing even more difficult. This mechanism causes a wheezing sound on exhaling.

Just to make things really clear from the beginning: *If your child develops an asthma attack or has any other difficulty breathing, you must call 9-1-1 or go to the ER immediately.* Use an inhaler, if you have one, while awaiting professional help.

Various homeopathic books talk about what can be done for asthma attack. That's all fine and good but do those things on the way to the ER. There's absolutely no reason whatsoever to neglect the need of your child to receive the most basic life resource: air.

Some children may present with frequent coughing or a prolonged cough that stays for weeks after what seems to be a simple cold. In all of these cases, you should consult your physician to make sure that you aren't missing the signs of asthma.

Conventional Treatment for Asthma

The mechanism of how things lead to the asthma attack is clear. What isn't clear is why some children have had asthma almost since they were one or two years old and why some haven't. Scientists pay a lot of attention to allergic reactions as the main reason for asthma. One of the main approaches used by allopathic medicine is suppression of allergic reactions in these children. The drugs they use are divided into two major groups:

1. *Relievers (bronchodilators):* These medications stop the spasms of the muscles in the airways. Currently used medications are sophisticated in both the design of the delivery system and efficacy. They provide very fast relief for an asthma attack. Unfortunately, some children who receive conventional long-term treatment also need to use this type of medication daily.

2. *Preventers:* These are medications used for long-term treatment. The best known from this group are the corticosteroid hormones. In some cases, these drugs are very efficacious and cause long-term remission of the illness. This is a temporary improvement. They don't cure the illness and are known to cause numerous very unpleasant side effects.

Most recently, two other major groups of medications have been introduced, *cromones* and *leukotriene receptor antagonists*. Cromones show better results in cases of mild asthma in children. Interestingly, the major side effect is a *bronchospasm*. Leukotriene receptor antagonists block the action of powerful *bronchioconstrictors*, called the leukotrienes. There are two main medications on the market, and only one of them, Montelukast (the generic name for Singulair), is approved for children younger than two. This group of medications is becoming increasingly popular. Unfortunately, it also has pretty serious side effects and does not offer a cure: just remission while the child is on the medication.

As you've probably noticed, the use of most of these medications in children younger than two years of age isn't recommended. So what can we do for the infants and toddlers? You may be familiar with the notion of allergy elimination. That's one approach. People also use herbal preparations with varying degrees of success. CAM modalities, such as acupuncture, Chinese and Tibetan medicine, and Ayurvedic medicine, may present good alternatives to conventional treatment.

Homeopathic Solutions

In treating asthma, I only have experience with homeopathy, and I must say that the results are very impressive. Certainly, the treatment is not always an easy proposition, like giving just one magic pellet, but success comes frequently enough to keep homeopaths busy treating plenty of children and adults with asthma.

A group of British homeopaths from the famous homeopathic hospital Glasgow Royal Infirmary conducted three series of studies on treatment of allergic asthma with homeopathically prepared allergens. They've been able to show reproducible success. Their most recent paper was published in 1994 in the *Lancet*.[5] They reported a study on twenty-eight patients with allergic asthma. The improvement after homeopathy appeared one week into treatment and held for eight weeks of follow-up. The effect of homeopathy was statistically better than placebo. They also performed the statistical analysis of all three studies (the current and two previous ones) and showed an even stronger benefit of homeopathy over placebo.

Research is an important part of trying to figure out what works and what does not. I believe that it's important to tell you the story of a little girl named Maria who developed asthma at one and a half, and whom I've known for seventeen years. This is the real story of a real person with a long follow-up. The majority of children cured from asthma disappear from the scope of my practice, as they should. Homeopathy gives them independence and happiness, and it obviously saves not only their lives but also a lot of money that otherwise would be spent on visits to the ER, doctors, and powerful drugs.

Maria and her family emigrated from the Dominican Republic soon after she turned one. She was a cute baby with round cheeks, who had a pleasant, mild disposition. She was a real trooper during the trip to America. Everything went well. Shortly after their arrival in New York, the family decided to celebrate. Maria loved chicken. Her parents normally would buy inexpensive chicken legs. On this occasion, they bought the most expensive chicken they could find. It wasn't organic, but it sure looked good! The very next day, Maria developed a rash in the folds of her skin. It was minor and her parents decided to wait to do anything. Otherwise she was healthy. The stress of their travels along with other factors, such as the hormones that I'm sure were contained in their chicken, had triggered a systemic response in Maria.

Maria did relatively well. But things got much worse when she had to go to school. She was given all the usual vaccines. Her parents had no choice. The rash turned out to be eczema, which got much worse, and soon she developed asthma. One night, she woke up having a serious asthma attack. It was so scary that her parents had to take her to the ER. For a few months after that, Maria had to use an inhaler, because frankly her parents couldn't figure out how to get homeopathic help for her. Then they called me.

There were many unique qualities about Maria. She was a sweet six-year-old who cried very easily. Maria was so shy, she spent most of our interview sitting on her mother's lap. Her mom told me that Maria wanted to be held each time she had an asthma attack, and she felt better if the window was wide open. Her mother complained that when Maria wasn't feeling well, she demanded all the attention she could get, wouldn't let go, and frequently asked her parents, "Do you love me?"

After asking many questions, I learned that Maria's asthma was worse at night. She only slept on her back and always stuck her feet out from under the covers. She didn't like to be in the sun. I also learned that the entire family was fascinated by the amount of butter this little girl could eat. She simply loved butter and ice cream. The combination of those symptoms pointed toward the homeopathic remedy *Pulsatilla nigricans*.

Pulsatilla would probably be the first thought of any homeopath reading this part of the story. Why? If you remember, in Chapter Eight, we spoke about keynote symptoms, the most characteristic symptoms of each remedy. On a rare occasion, a child comes to the homeopath's office with a severe, seemingly incurable problem, but the picture of the remedy is very clear. The striking features of Maria's presentation were in the mental area. These included her sweetness and her need for attention on the one hand and her shyness on the other. In general characteristics, she was remarkably worse at night, was very warm, slept on her back, and also craved ice cream and butter.

Although they would have been useless for a conventional physician, these data clearly spoke to me, a homeopath, in the language of *Pulsatilla*. The emerging quality of the virtual *Pulsatilla* person was obvious to me in Maria's case, as it would be to anyone else who studied homeopathy and had successfully prescribed this remedy. Still I had to dot all the i's and cross all the t's by asking many specific questions to make sure that there was no alternative to this, my original choice.

The type of eczema she had, and the fact that Maria had been brought in by her parents to address the main complaint of asthma, also helped me make a solid choice. I certainly wanted to prescribe a remedy that was known from the provings to cause these problems and that's known from two hundred years of homeopathic practice to cure these ailments. Looking up for just two of these things showed the following results. *Pulsatilla* is one of 304 remedies that can be helpful for asthma. In addition, it is one of the sixteen in this group that are most frequently indicated. It is also one of 161 remedies listed in the *Repertory* under the rubric *eczema*. Finally, I felt confident. I prescribed *Pulsatilla*.

I want to remind you that there are very many homeopathic remedies for asthma. There's no one magic pill. So don't rush out and give this same remedy to your child. You need to consult with a homeopath. Even if this picture seems similar to your child's, remember that I had to look for the symptoms. I know what to look for, and my repertoire is much larger than just a few remedies. If any of the symptoms had indicated even a slight possibility of a different remedy, I would have been able to conduct a full and thorough investigation, because I know these other remedies, not only *Pulsatilla*.

Maria got better. In a few short weeks, she didn't have wheezing anymore. Her eczema got a little bit worse and then it disappeared. A few times throughout the years since then, she's had to take a repeat dose of the same remedy, but overall she has done extremely well. She's never needed an inhaler since. I am talking about at least ten years of leading an asthma-free life. She also has been able to stay allergy-free around the family dog, and they still have a cat at home that spends most of his time sitting on Maria's lap.

Obesity

The same thing has been said about other illnesses discussed in this book, but I'll have to say it again. Obesity is reaching epidemic proportions in the United States. As a matter of fact, the term *epidemic* is widely used in reports on both adult and childhood obesity.

Over the past three decades, we've watched an enormous increase in the number of children suffering from chronic obesity. The rate of this condition has more than doubled in the age groups two to five and twelve to nineteen, and it has more than tripled among children age six to eleven. It's estimated that nine million children older than six are presently obese. According to the 2003 U.S. Census, we had 53.3 million children age five to seventeen. Nine million is therefore a truly significant proportion.

Certainly, reading about a recent American Heart Association report would make any parent of young children anxious. This headline was printed from an Associated Press story on December 30, 2004: "The obesity epidemic is reaching down to the playpen: More than 10 percent of U.S. children ages 2 to 5 are overweight."

Some highlights of the American Heart Association report are the following:

- About one million youths ages twelve to nineteen in the United States—or 4.2 percent of the age group—have *metabolic syndrome*, defined as three or more of the following five factors: high triglycerides, low "good" cholesterol, high blood sugar, high blood pressure, and a big waistline. These factors raise the risk of heart disease.
- In 2002, heart disease killed 927,448 Americans, keeping its place as the nation's number-one killer.
- The Framingham Study found that being overweight or obese could take years off your life. For example, a forty-year-old woman who does not smoke could lose 3.3 years of life because she is overweight and 7.1 years for being obese.

I don't think we need to repeat too many statistics, as everyone already knows that our children are becoming heavier. A few simple reasons for that are the following:

- More and more children live in cities and suburbs where walking and other physical activities are discouraged by the design and the lifestyle.
- There's an increased consumption of fast food, which is high in calories and fat.
- There's a decrease in physical activities at school and after school. Children are usually driven to and from school. After school, the time that previous generations spent running around in the outdoors is now used for watching TV, surfing the Internet, and playing video games.

In September 2004, the Institute of Medicine of the National Academies published a fact sheet entitled "Childhood Obesity in the United States: Facts and Figures."[6] It talks about the significant physical and emotional consequences of this illness and concludes that preventing childhood obesity should become a national priority. According to this report, being obese may lead to low self-esteem, negative body image, and depression.

As a homeopath and a psychiatrist, I frequently have to deal with weight problems in my patients. From the holistic perspective, obesity can have a number of sources: notably, overeating and lack of exercise. The solution seems simple: eat less and exercise more. Here are a few other possible steps to consider that Andrew Weil, M.D., suggests on his Web site:

- *Curb screen time.* Limit the time your child spends watching television, sitting at the computer, or playing video games.

- *Set a good example.* Studies have found that children are more likely to be physically active if their parents and siblings are active and if they're encouraged to take part in physical activities. Take family walks, hikes, or bike rides on a daily basis, if possible.

- *Emphasize nutritious foods.* Don't limit the amount your child eats, but make sure the foods your child does eat are low in fat and high in fiber. When making these changes, say that you're doing it for the entire family to avoid drawing attention to your child's need to lose weight.

- *Eat meals together.* Family breakfasts and dinners give you more control over what your child eats and allow you to make sure that everyone gets at least two nutritious meals per day.

- *Think about drinks.* Substitute for fruit juices, sodas, and whole milk. Drinks can provide a surprisingly large number of calories per day.

- *Teach a relaxation technique.* If your child eats in response to stress, you might show her how a relaxation technique, such as deep breathing, can help her calm down.[7]

Dealing with obesity has to be directed to achieving two goals:

- *Prevention.* Homeopathy can be an important part of these efforts. By eliminating the need to take conventional medications that are known to cause weight gain, such as hormones and antipsychotic medications, homeopathy helps to significantly decrease the number of obese children.

- *Treatment.* Some children who are seemingly healthy still have a tendency to eat more than they need to and to become overweight. Constitutional treatment of these children addresses their core issues and ultimately helps resolve this problem, too.

Unfortunately, I cannot give you the name of a remedy for obesity that's going to solve every contributing issue. Clearly, children who have significant weight problems caused either by a medication or by insulin-dependent diabetes, will be less likely to see benefits from homeopathy. These problems are also rising among children.

Of course, we also need to accept that there are children who are naturally big. However, this doesn't mean they have to be obese. Rational eating habits and exercise can make children strong and fit no matter what their innate structure and size are. Regardless of the modality used, these two factors remain the foundation of successful treatment of this issue.

The Homeopathic Approach

Let's see how homeopathy works for one obese child, named Frank, who had a large appetite. By the time I saw him, Frank was six and going strong. He ate a lot. He also had a tendency to like sweets. Actually, his weight, although an issue, wasn't the main reason his parents brought him to see me. They were concerned that their son simply couldn't stop eating, especially at night.

Trying to stop Frank from eating practically nonstop in the evenings had become like a family sport. He had an older sister who didn't have a weight problem. So the three of them—Frank's mother, father, and older sister, Ann—were the opposing "team." It was simply ridiculous. Frank would find various reasons to be in the kitchen and go hunting for sweets. They tried banning sweets from the house, but it caused so much distress for Frankie, that they decided not to "torture" him. Poor boy.

A pediatrician suggested giving Frank a thorough workup to make sure that he didn't have problems with his thyroid gland or diabetes. Everything seemed to be OK for the time being. Luckily for all of us, when they brought him to see me, this little boy had many very prominent symptoms that quickly led me to prescribe the homeopathic remedy *Lycopodium*. Of course, I had to make sure that the remedy I gave him would help him with both increased appetite and obesity. In Frank's case, obesity was probably a result of a literally ravenous appetite. As previously noted, his appetite increased mostly at night. This information was very important to me, because it allowed me to narrow down my search.

Let's go through the steps of the search together. There are 137 remedies that can be helpful for obesity. *Lycopodium* is one of them. Two hundred and thirty-six remedies can be helpful for increased appetite, but only twenty-three in this group mollify an appetite that increases mainly at night. *Lycopodium* is one of them. To ensure we're on the right track now, we must combine this rubric *obesity* in the *Repertory* with the rubric *ravenous appetite at night*. This one has twenty remedies in it. One is *Lycopodium*.

Imagine that we've boiled down the search to twenty or twenty-three remedies only. Still, we need to find the one and only remedy that will truly help. We need to find more symptoms that are unique to Frank. Another interesting thing was that he *loved* sweets; he absolutely felt he couldn't live without them. There are 151 remedies that can help with this issue, and *Lycopodium* is one of the eight most prominent in the group.

Even though everything is looking good for *Lycopodium*, to a homeopath at this stage of searching, it's still just a possibility. If we cross-referenced the symptoms collected so far, they wouldn't be good enough. We need to identify at least one more symptom in Frank that's also very characteristic of the remedy. That might help narrow down our possibilities even further.

It turned out that I had more than one more important symptom to work with in Frank's case. First, he was morbidly afraid of speaking in front of other people. The cross-reference with this symptom still leaves us with twenty-two possible remedies. Second, Frank also felt full all the time and had a lot of gas. Although this group contains over 270 remedies, cross-referenced with the other three groups of symptoms we're using leaves us with only twenty possibilities. An experienced homeopath can look at these choices and see which ones are still viable and which need to be eliminated from the list of candidates. This short evaluation already leaves us with only ten choices.

During the interview, I noticed that Frank was arrogant with his parents and nice with me. I asked about this behavior and his parents informed me that their son was the sweetest boy on earth when he was at school and a tyrant at home. Again, this information reminded me of the picture of *Lycopodium*—it is a very characteristic symptom of the remedy.

But I needed more precision. It turned out that Frank really hated mornings and that he only liked warm drinks and food. He also happened to sleep only on his right side. Any of these symptoms taken alone would not confirm *Lycopodium* as my first choice, but taken in combination, a picture of the remedy definitely emerged.

Just to give you a glimpse of how fine the distinctions between remedies sometimes are, another homeopathic remedy, *Sulphur*, that could have been a possibility for Frank was eliminated after I learned that Frank hated everything cold. People needing *Sulphur* are frequently very thirsty for cold drinks, and they are rarely shy, either.

I am sure that some of my readers, especially those who decided to jump to this chapter without reading the rest of the book, are now standing by the door ready to go buy *Lycopodium* in order to begin their journey to become a lean, mean, beautiful machine themselves, in addition to giving this remedy to their children. If you're one of them, please come back to your chair and read the beginning of the book. *Lycopodium* is just one of many homeopathic remedies that can be helpful with obesity.

As with all other remedies (and many conventional medications), we don't understand why this remedy works. What we can say for sure is that as a result of its action in people who exhibit the right signs and symptoms, it helps reset the endocrine, immune, central nervous, and digestive systems—just to name a few. This action leads to normalization of appetite, disappearance of bloating, weight loss, and changes on the emotional level that remove a constant need to fulfill psychological emptiness and the feeling of inferiority that many overeaters have. That much we know.

Two months after our first appointment, Frank's parents were happy to report a significant decrease in their son's appetite, especially at night. A few months later, he was able to maintain a fairly normal food intake regimen. He also started playing more sports with his father and his friends. Life was going well for Frank.

Then Frank and I had a long break. The next time I saw him was almost a year and a half later for an entirely different problem. He was so much thinner that I could barely recognize him. I don't know what his situation is today. He got better and didn't need me anymore, so he hasn't been in for a visit.

I've seen numerous cases of obesity. The rule of thumb in this type of situation is this: if the appropriate remedy is clear, and if the child isn't taking any medications that would cause weight gain and also doesn't have severe endocrine problems, the results of homeopathy could be simply excellent—provided the child exercises, that is. Movement and sensible eating are requirements for fitness. No remedy can substitute for that.

Conclusion

I hope that someday soon someone will discover the active mechanism behind the two hundred–yearlong success of homeopathic remedies. No doubt, this individual will receive a Nobel Prize and the rest of us will be empowered to lead much healthier, happier lives.

Appendix A: Active Concentrations of Various Homeopathic Potencies

In order to be an informed partner in your children's medical care, you may find yourself wondering how strong the potentized remedies a homeopath has prescribed are and how much active substance remains in them. A quick scan of the following chart will reveal several important facts about a remedy's preparation, including its degree of dilution, how many succussions have been performed, and how much substance remains.

As you can plainly see, at 24X and 12C, the original ingredient is no longer detectable. It's obvious that even at the lowest potencies (for example, 3C or 6X), remedies are extremely safe because there is so little original substance in them. You'll notice, however, that the number of succussions differs between these two potencies. In practice, 24X is actually never used. The main point of interest in this chart is that the higher the dilution, the more succussions have been performed, which, according to homeopathic theory and practice, makes the remedy more potent and longer acting. (See Table A.1.)

Table A.1. Potentized Remedies: Strength and Amount of Active Substance.

X Potencies	Number of Successions	Attenuation	C Potencies	Number of Successions	Amount of the Original Ingredient in 1 Gram of the Final Product
1X	10	10^1			100mg
2X	20	10^2	1C	10	10mg
3X	30	10^3			1mg
4X	40	10^4	2C	20	100µg
5X	50	10^5			10µg
6X	60	10^6	3C	30	1µg
7X	70	10^7			100ng
8X	80	10^8	4C	40	10ng
9X	90	10^9			1ng
10X	100	10^{10}	5C	50	100pg
11X	110	10^{11}			10pg
12X	120	10^{12}	6C	60	1pg
24X	240	10^{24}	12C	120	Undetectable
60X	600	10^{60}	30C	300	
400X	4,000	10^{400}	200C	2,000	
		$10^{2,000}$	1M	10,000	
		$10^{20,000}$	10M	100,000	
		$10^{100,000}$	50M	500,000	
		$10^{200,000}$	CM	1,000,000	
		$10^{2,000,000}$	MM	2,000,000	

Appendix B: Selection from *Homeopathic Materia Medica* by William Boericke, M.D.

We've spoken many times about the *Materia Medica*, the main source of information about remedies. The following chapter, on the frequently prescribed remedy *Calcarea carbonica*, is reproduced from a famous edition. I have a copy in my office. A high-quality book, it clearly shows the wear and tear of frequent use. The only book in my office that has more wear is my copy of Kent's *Repertory*, which by now has no front jacket. Before computer programs, homeopaths all repertorized by hand and read *Materia Medica* from books. Boericke's is a concise version of a fuller *Materia Medica*.

A few facts illustrate how different volumes of *Materia Medica* can be. One of the most recent books by Frans Vermeulen has seventeen single-spaced pages dedicated to symptoms of *Calcarea carbonica*. Overall, this remedy can be helpful with 10,860 symptoms! Obviously, it is a major polychrest. Of course, an untrained reader cannot help but get lost trying to figure out what remedy to give. A simple list of symptoms has no life. A homeopath has a clear image in mind of a virtual person who represents *Calcarea carbonica*. There are many details, yet the major characteristics always remain the same. This kind of knowledge comes only with years of study and experience.

Calcarea Carbonica: also known as carbonate of lime

This great Hahnemannian anti-psoric is a constitutional remedy *par excellence*. Its chief action is centered in the vegetative sphere, impaired nutrition being the keynote of its action, the glands, skin, and bones, being instrumental in the changes wrought. Increased local and general perspiration, swelling of glands, scrofulous and rachitic conditions generally offer numerous opportunities for the exhibition of Calcarea. Incipient phthisis (*Ars jod; Tuberculin*). It covers the tickling cough, fleeting chest pains, nausea, acidity and dislike of fat. Gets out of breath easily. *A jaded state, mental or physical, due to overwork. Abscesses in deep muscles; polypi and exostoses.* Pituitary and thyroid disfunction.

Raised blood coagulability (*Strontium*). Is a definite stimulant to the periosteum. Is a hæmostatic and gives this power probably to the gelatine injections.

Easy relapses, interrupted convalescence. Persons of scrofulous type, who take cold easily, with increased mucous secretions, children who grow fat, are large-bellied, with large head, pale skin, chalky look, the so-called leuco-phlegmatic temperament; affections caused by working in water. Great sensitiveness to cold; partial sweats. Children crave eggs and eat dirt and other indigestible things; are prone to diarrhœa. Calcarea patient is fat, fair, flabby and perspiring and cold, damp and sour.

Mind. *Apprehensive*; worse towards evening; *fears loss of reason, misfortune*, contagious diseases. *Forgetful*, confused, low-spirited. Anxiety with palpitation. Obstinacy; slight mental effort produces hot head. Averse to work or exertion.

Head. Sense of weight on top of head. Headache, with cold hands and feet. Vertigo on ascending, and when turning head. Headache from overlifting, from mental exertion, with nausea. Head feels hot and heavy, with pale face. *Icy coldness in, and on the head*, especially right side. Open fontanelles; head enlarged; *much perspiration, wets the pillow*. Itching of the scalp. Scratches head on waking.

Eyes. Sensitive to light. Lachrymation in open air and early in morning. *Spots and ulcers on cornea.* Lachrymal ducts closed from exposure to cold. Easy fatigue of eyes. Far sighted. Itching of lids, swollen, scurfy. *Chronic dilatation of pupils.* Cataract. Dimness of vision, as if looking through a mist. Lachrymal fistula; scrofulous ophthalmia.

Ears. Throbbing; cracking in ears; stitches; pulsating pain as if something would press out. Deafness from working in water. Polypi which bleed easily. Scrofulous inflammation *with muco-purulent otorrhœa, and enlarged glands.* Perversions of hearing; hardness of hearing. Eruption on and behind ear (*Petrol*). Cracking noises in ear. Sensitive to cold about ears and neck.

Nose. Dry, *nostrils sore, ulcerated.* Stoppage of nose, also with fetid, yellow discharge. Offensive odor in nose. *Polypi*; swelling at root of nose. Epistaxis. Coryza. *Takes cold at every change of weather.* Catarrhal symptoms with hunger; coryza alternates with colic.

Face. Swelling of upper lip. Pale, with deep-seated eyes, surrounded by dark rings. Crusta lactea; itching, burning after washing. Submaxillary glands swollen. Goitre. Itching of pimples in whiskers. Pain from right mental foramen along lower jaw to ear.

Mouth. Persistent *sour taste.* Mouth fills with sour water. Dryness of tongue at night. Bleeding of gums. Difficult and delayed dentition. Teeth ache; excited by current of air, anything cold or hot. Offensive smell from mouth. Burning pain at tip of tongue; worse, anything warm taken into stomach.

Throat. *Swelling of tonsils* and submaxillary glands; stitches on swallowing. Hawking-up of mucus. Difficult swallowing. *Goitre.* Parotid fistula.

Stomach. Aversion to meat, boiled things; craving for indigestible things-chalk, coal, pencils; also for eggs, salt and sweets. Milk disagrees. Frequent sour eructations; sour vomiting. Dislike of fat. Loss of appetite when overworked. Heartburn and loud belching.

Cramps in stomach; worse, pressure, cold water. Ravenous hunger. Swelling over pit of stomach, like a saucer turned bottom up. Repugnance to hot food. Pain in epigastric region to touch. Thirst; longing for cold drinks. Aggravation while eating. Hyperchlorhydria (Phos).

Abdomen. Sensitive to slightest pressure. Liver region painful when stooping. Cutting in abdomen; swollen abdomen. Incarcerated flatulence. *Inguinal and mesenteric glands swollen* and painful. Cannot bear tight clothing around the waist. *Distention* with hardness. *Gallstone colic.* Increase of fat in abdomen. Umbilical hernia. Trembling; weakness, as if sprained. Children are late in learning to walk.

Stool. Crawling and constriction in rectum. Stool large and hard (*Bry*); whitish, watery, *sour.* Prolapse ani, and burning, stinging hæmorrhoids. Diarrhœa of undigested, food, fetid, with ravenous appetite. *Children's diarrhœa.* Constipation; stool at first hard, then pasty, then liquid.

Urine. Dark, brown, sour, fetid, abundant, with white sediment, bloody. Irritable bladder. Enuresis (Use 30th, also *Tuberculin.* 1 *m.*).

Male. *Frequent emissions.* Increased desire. Semen emitted too soon. Coition followed by weakness and irritability.

Female. Before menses, headache, colic, chilliness and leucorrhœa. Cutting pains in uterus during menstruation. Menses *too early, too profuse, too long,* with vertigo, toothache and *cold, damp feet*; the least excitement causes their return. Uterus easily displaced. Leucorrhœa, *milky* (*Sepia*). Burning and itching of parts before and after menstruation; in little girls. Increased sexual desire; easy conception. Hot swelling breasts. Breasts tender and swollen before menses. Milk too abundant; disagreeable to child. Deficient lactation, with distended breasts in lymphatic women. Much sweat about external genitals. Sterility with copious menses. Uterine polypi.

Respiratory. Tickling cough troublesome at night, dry and free expectoration in morning; cough when playing piano, or by eating.

Persistent, irritating cough from arsenical wall paper (Clarke). Extreme dyspnœa. *Painless hoarseness*; worse in the morning. Expectoration only during the day; thick, yellow, sour mucus. Bloody expectoration; with sour sensation in chest. *Suffocating spells*; tightness, burning and soreness in chest; *worse going upstairs* or slightest ascent, must sit down. Sharp pains in chest from before backwards. *Chest very sensitive to touch, percussion, or pressure.* Longing for fresh air. Scanty, salty expectoration (*Lyc*).

Heart. Palpitation at night and after eating. Palpitation with feeling of coldness, with restless oppression of chest; after suppressed eruption.

Back. Pain as if sprained; can scarcely rise; from overlifting. Pain between shoulder-blades, impeding breathing. Rheumatism in lumbar region; weakness in small of back. Curvature of dorsal vertebræ. Nape of neck stiff and rigid. *Renal colic.*

Extremities. Rheumatoid pains, as after exposure to wet. Sharp sticking, as if parts were wrenched or sprained. *Cold, damp* feet; feel as if damp stockings were worn. Cold knees cramps in calves. Sour foot-sweat. Weakness of extremities. Swelling of joints, especially knee. Burning of soles of feet. Sweat of hands. Arthritic nodosities. *Soles of feet raw.* Feet feel cold and dead at night. Old sprains. Tearing in muscles.

Sleep. Ideas crowding in her mind prevent sleep. Horrid visions when opening eyes. Starts at every noise; fears that she will go crazy. Drowsy in early part of evening. Frequent waking at night. *Same disagreeable idea always arouses from light slumber.* Night terrors (*Kali phos*). Dreams of the dead.

Fever. *Chill at 2 pm begins internally in stomach region. Fever with sweat.* Pulse full and frequent. Chilliness and heat. Partial sweats. *Night sweats, especially on head,* neck and chest. Hectic fever. Heat at night during menstruation, with restless sleep. *Sweat over head in children, so that pillow becomes wet.*

Skin. Unhealthy; readily ulcerating; flaccid. Small wounds do not heal readily. Glands swollen. Nettle rash; better in cold air. Warts on face and hands. *Petechial eruptions.* Chilblains. Boils.

Modalities. *Worse,* from exertion, mental or physical; ascending; *cold* in every form; water, washing, moist air, wet weather; during full moon; standing. *Better,* dry climate and weather; lying on painful side. Sneezing (pain in head and nape).

Relationship. Antidotes: *Camph; Ipec; Nit ac; Nux.* Complementary: Bell; Rhus; Lycop; Silica.

Calcar is useful after Sulphur where the pupils remain dilated. When Pulsatilla failed in school girls.

Incompatible: *Bry*; Sulphur should not be given *after* Calc.

Compare: *Aqua calcar.* Lime-water (1/2 teaspoonful in milk); (as injection for oxyuris vermicularis), and *Calc caust*—slaked lime— (pain in back and heels, jaws and malar bones; also symptoms of influenza). *Calc brom* (removes inflammatory products from uterus; children of lax fiber, nervous and irritable, with gastric and cerebral irritation. *Tendency to brain disease.* Insomnia and cerebral congestion. Give 1x trituration). *Sulph* (differs in being worse by heat, hot feet, etc).

Calcar calcinata-Calcined oyster-shell-a remedy for warts. Use 3d trituration. *Calcarea ovorum. Ova tosta*-Toasted egg-shells (*backache and leucorrhœa.* Feeling as if back were broken in two; tired feeling. Also effective in controlling suffering from cancer).

Calcar lactic (anæmias, hæmophilia, urticaria, where the coagulability of the blood is diminished; nervous headache with œdema of eyelids, lips or hands; 15 grains three times a day, but low potencies often equally effective).

Calcar lacto-phosph (5 grains 3 times a day in cyclic vomiting and migraine).

Calc mur. Calcium chloratum-Rademacher's Liquor (1 part to 2 of distilled water, of which take 15 drops in half a cup of water, five times daily. Boils. *Porrigo capitis. Vomiting of all food and drink,* with gastric pain. Impetigo, glandular swellings, angioneurotic œdema. Pleurisy with effusion. Eczema in infants).

Calcar picrata, (peri-follicular inflammation; a remedy of prime importance in *recurring or chronic boils,* particularly when located on parts thinly covered with muscle tissue, as on shinbones, coccyx, *auditory canal,* dry, scurfy accumulation and exfoliation of epithelial scales, etc, styes, phlyctenules. Use 3x trit).

Compare also with Calcarea; Lycop; Silica; Pulsat; Chamom.

Dose. Sixth trit. Thirtieth and higher potencies. Should not be repeated too frequently in elderly people.[1]

Appendix C: Selection from *Repertory of the Homeopathic Materia Medica* by James Tyler Kent

Repertory is a cross-reference tool used by homeopaths to evaluate the patient as a whole person. It is divided into over thirty chapters, most corresponding to parts of the human body. Some chapters, such as Mind, Generalities, Fever, Perspiration, and Vision, describe something other than an organ. Modern versions contain two thousand–plus pages.

Today the majority of homeopaths use sophisticated computerized repertories that allow them fast access to the rubrics they need, as well as offering them a few ways of cross-referencing and analyzing the data. Prominent American homeopath David Kent Warkentin designed the first program of this type, Mac Repertory. In my practice, I use RADAR, a program that appeared later. Both systems, and a few others like them, are popular. They offer similar core information with various menus of additional options. They also include large, fully searchable libraries of homeopathic books and journals.

In the following reproduction, you can see that we are in a chapter entitled Mind. After the name of the rubric, many abbreviations of the names of homeopathic remedies are provided in alphabetical order. These are remedies that either caused this symptom during a proving or frequently cure this symptom—or both.

Mind

SADNESS, mental depression: *Abies-n.*, abrot., acal., acet-ac., **Acon.**, act-sp., *aesc.*, agar., *agn.*, ail., all-c., aloe., *alum.*, alumn., *am-c.*, *am-m.*, *ambr.*, ammc., *anac.*, anan., *ant-c.*, apis., apoc., aran., *arg-m.*, *arg-n.*, *arn.*, **Ars-i.**, **Ars.**, arum-t., *asaf.*, asar., aster., **Aur-m.**, aur-s., **Aur.**, bapt., *bar-c.*, *bar-m.*, *bell.*, benz-ac., berb., bol., bov., *brom.*, *bry.*, *bufo.*, *cact.*, calad., **Calc-ar.**, *calc-f.*, *calc-p.*, **Calc-s.**, **Calc.**, *camph.*, cann-i., *cann-s.*, *canth.*, *caps.*, **Carb-an.**, **Carb-s.**, *carb-v.*, card-m., carl., cast., **Caust.**, **Cham.**, *chel.*, *chin-a.*, *chin-s.*, **Chin.**, *cic.*, **Cimic.**, cina., cinnb., *clem.*, cob., coca., *cocc.*, coch., *coff.*, *colch.*, *coloc.*, *con.*, *corn.*, *croc.*, **Crot-c.**, *crot-h.*, crot-t., *cupr.*, *cur.*, *cycl.*, *dig.*, *dros.*, *dulc.*, echi., elaps., eug., eup-per., eup-pur., eupho., euphr., *ferr-ar.*, **Ferr-i.**, *ferr-p.*, **Ferr.**, fl-ac., gamb., **Gels.**, glon., **Graph.**, *grat.*, guai., haem., ham., **Hell.**, *helon.*, hep., **Hipp.**, *hura.*, *hydr.*, hydrc., *hyos.*, hyper., **Ign.**, Ind., *indg.*, **Iod.**, *ip.*, iris., *kali-ar.*, kali-bi., **Kali-br.**, *kali-c.*, kali-chl., *kali-i.*, kali-n., **Kali-p.**, kali-s., kalm., kreos., **Lac-c.**, *lac-d.*, **Lach.**, lachn., lact., lam., *laur.*, lec., **Lept.**, **Lil-t.**, lob., **Lyc.**, lycps., mag-c., mag-m., mag-s., *manc.*, *mang.*, med., meny., *merc-c.*, *merc-i-r.*, **Merc.**, merl., **Mez.**, mosch., *mur-ac.*, **Murx.**, *mygal.*, myric., *naja.*, **Nat-a.**, **Nat-c.**, **Nat-m.**, *nat-p.*, **Nat-s.**, nicc., **Nit-ac.**, nux-m., *nux-v.*, *ol-an.*, olnd., op., oxyt., *petr.*, *ph-ac.*, phel., *phos.*, *phyt.*, pic-ac., plan., **Plat.**, *plb.*, podo., prun-s., **Psor.**, ptel., **Puls.**, ran-s., raph., rheum., rhod., **Rhus-t.**, *rhus-v.*, rob., rumx., *ruta.*, sabad., sabin., sang., sanic., sarr., sars., sec., senec., seneg., **Sep.**, sil., *spig.*, *spong.*, **Stann.**, staph., *still.*, *stram.*, stront., *stry.*, *sul-ac.*, **Sulph.**, *tab.*, tarent., tell., ter., **Thuj.**, til., tril., uran., ust., valer., *verat-v.*, **Verat.**, verb., vib., viol-t., *visc.*, xan., **Zinc.**, zing., ziz.

daytime: Agn., ant-c., dros., nat-m., phel., stann., sul-ac., sulph., zinc.

morning: Agar., aloe., *alum.*, alumn., am-c., anac., ant-c., apis., arg-m., arg-n., *aur.*, bar-c., bar-m., calad., calc., cann-i., canth., *carb-an.*, cast., caust., con., cop., dulc., graph., hep., hura., hyper., kali-c., kali-p., kali-s., kreos., **Lach.**, *lyc.*, mag-m., mag-p., mag-s., manc., mur-ac., naja., *nat-s.*, nicc., *nit-ac.*, *nux-v.*, ol-an., op., *petr.*, *phos.*, *plat.*, plb., *puls.*, rhus-t., sarr., sars., sep., sil., sul-ac., sulph., tarax., zinc.[1]

Notes

Introduction

1. S. Hahnemann, *Materia Medica Pura* (New Delhi, India: B. Jain Publishers, Reprint edition 1999), Volume 2, p. 2.
2. J. Winston, *The Faces of Homeopathy* (Tawa, New Zealand: Great Auk Publishing, 1999), p. 31.
3. Ibid.
4. Ibid., p. 216.
5. Ibid., pp. 316–317.

Chapter One

1. The terms *homeopathic medicine* and *allopathic medicine* were both invented by Hahnemann. In Greek, *homeo* means "the same." *Allo* means "different."
2. Yellow jasmine is not to be confused with real yellow jasmine from Madeira. It's actually woodbine, not a true jasmine.

Chapter Two

1. M. Quinn, "Homeopathic Pharmacy." In *Classical Homeopathy*, M. Carlston, ed. (Philadelphia: Churchill Livingstone, 2003), p. 150.
2. As you may have figured out already, the number in front of letter C multiplied by 2 will indicate the exact dilution of the remedy. For 12C, for example, $12 \times 2 = 24$ (dilution is 10^{24} times).

3. Avogadro's number (6.023×10^{23}) is the number of molecules contained in one mole of a substance. One molecule of a remedy substance in a mole is approximately equivalent to 24X (12C) dilution level. In other words, mathematical calculations show that not one molecule of the original substance can be found in a homeopathic remedy at the 24X (12C) dilution level. This explanation is taken from J. Yasgur, *Yasgur's Homeopathic Dictionary and Holistic Health Reference* (Greenville, Penn.: Vann Hoy, 1998), p. 25.

4. What is the theoretical maximum content of *Arsenicum album* 6X in a hundred grams of the final product (let's say in drops, for example)? One microgram, or 0.000001 (one millionth) of a gram. The toxic dose of *Arsenicum album* is one milligram per kilogram. So for a ten-kilogram child (approximately twenty-two pounds), the toxic dose would be ten milligrams. To produce this amount, we'd have to give the child 2.2 pounds (a thousand grams) of *Arsenicum album* 6X. The number of toxic doses in the container for this remedy is 1/1,000. This means that even if the child consumes a hundred grams of *Arsenicum album* 6X, nothing bad is going to happen.

In real life, a container with homeopathic pellets in it holds significantly less than a hundred grams of medication because most of the pellet is milk sugar, which makes homeopathic remedies totally safe. By comparison, a bottle of a hundred tablets of acetaminophen, a commonly prescribed painkiller, contains twenty toxic doses for a twenty-two-pound child (ten kilograms), which means it holds two thousand more toxic doses than the container of *Arsenicum album* 6X.

Actually, this is a purely hypothetical situation, as the majority of homeopathic remedies are rarely used at attenuations lower than 6C, which equals one picogram (0.000000000001 gram) concentration per one hundred grams of the final product, or higher.

Chapter Four

1. A *placebo* is an inactive substance, containing no medicine, which is commonly referred to as a "sugar pill." Used as a control in clinical trials of medications, it looks, smells, and tastes just like the drug that's being tested.
2. A. G. Johnson, "Surgery as Placebo," *Lancet* 344, no. 8930 (1994): 1140–1142.
3. J. Kleijnen, P. Knipschild, and G. ter Riet, "Clinical Trials of Homoeopathy," *British Medical Journal* 302 (February 9, 1991): 316–323.

    K. Linde et al., "Are the Clinical Effects of Homeopathy Placebo Effects? A Meta-analysis of Placebo-Controlled Trials," *Lancet* 350, no. 9081 (September 20, 1997): 834–843.
4. D. Eskinazi, D.D.S., Ph.D., "Homeopathy Re-revisited: Is Homeopathy Compatible with Biomedical Observations?" *Archives of Internal Medicine* 159 (September 1999): 1981–1987.
5. W. B. Jonas, "Do Homeopathic Nosodes Protect Against Infection? An Experimental Test," *Alternative Therapies in Health and Medicine* 5, no. 5 (September 1999): 36–40.
6. D. Castro and G. G. Nogueira, "Use of the Nosode Meningococcinum as a Preventive Against Meningitis," *Journal of American Institute of Homeopathy* 68 (1975): 211–219.
7. S. Hahnemann, *Organon of the Medical Art*, W. B. O'Reilly, trans. (Palo Alto, Calif.: Birdcage Press, 2001), paragraph 273.
8. E. Bach, as cited in J. Winston, *The Faces of Homeopathy*, p. 187.

Chapter Five

1. A *polychrest* is a remedy whose provings and clinical applications show that it has many widespread uses, covering a wide variety of mental, emotional, and physical symptomatology.

Yasgur's Homeopathic Dictionary and Holistic Health Reference, 191. A *small remedy* is a remedy with few symptoms. This doesn't mean that the remedy is rarely used. It just means that the remedy is known to elicit few symptoms, Ibid., 236.

Chapter Eight

1. Autism statistics are available from Fighting Autism, an education and advocacy organization based in Gibsonia, Penn. Web site: www.fightingautism.org.
2. C. T. Gordon, "Psychopharmacological Treatments for Symptoms and Behaviors in Autism Spectrum Disorder," *Advocate: The Newsletter of The Autism Society of America* 33 (2000): 28–31.
3. FDA Public Health Advisory, "Suicidality in Children and Adolescents Being Treated with Antidepressant Medications" (October 15, 2004). Web site: www.fda.gov/cder/drug/antidepressants/SSRIPHA200410.htm.

Chapter Nine

1. An anaphylactic reaction is a severe, rapid, and sometimes fatal allergic reaction to a given substance (commonly a vaccine, penicillin, shellfish, or insect venom) to which someone has become sensitized by previous exposure.
2. M. A. Taylor et al., "Randomised Controlled Trial of Homeopathy Versus Placebo in Perennial Allergic Rhinitis with Overview of Four Trial Series," *British Medical Journal* 321 (2000): 471–476.
3. D. Reilly et al., "Is Homoeopathy a Placebo Response? Controlled Trial of Homoeopathic Potency, with Pollen in Hay Fever as Model," *Lancet* 2 (1986): 881–886.
4. Allergy statistics are taken from University of Maryland Medicine. Web site: www.umm.edu/allergies/stats.htm.
5. D. Reilly et al., "Is Evidence for Homoeopathy Reproducible?" *Lancet* 344, no. 8937 (1994): 1601–1606.

6. "Childhood Obesity in the United States: Facts and Figures," Institute of Medicine of the National Academies (2004). Web site: www.iom.edu/Object.File/Master/22/606/0.pdf.
7. Suggestions for weight control are taken from Dr. Andrew Weil's Web site (2005). Web site: www.drweil.com/u/HC/HCA210/#14.

Appendix B

1. W. Boericke, *Pocket Manual of Homeopathic Materia Medica and Repertory* (New Delhi, India: B. Jain Publishers Pvt. Ltd., Reprint Edition 2002 [Original edition 1906]), pp. 144–148.

Appendix C

1. J. T. Kent, *Repertory of the Homoeopathic Materia Medica* (Sitting Bourne, Kent, UK: Homocopathic Book Service, 1990 [Original edition 1912]), p. 75.

Suggested Reading

Bellavite, P., M.D., and Signorini, A., M.D. *The Emerging Science of Homeopathy.* Berkeley: North Atlantic Books, 2002.

Boericke, W. *Pocket Manual of Homeopathic Materia Medica and Repertory.* New Delhi, India: B. Jain Publishers, Reprint Edition 2002 (Original Edition 1906).

Borneman, J. P. "The Mortar and Pestle: Homeopathic Nosodes—Are They Useful for Bioterrorism?" *Homeopathy Today* (December 2001).

Carlston, M., ed. *Classical Homeopathy.* London: Churchill Livingstone, 2002.

Castro, D., and Nogueira, G. G. "Use of the Nosode Meningococcinum as a Preventive Against Meningitis." *Journal of American Institute of Homeopathy* 68 (1975).

Dooley, T., N.D., M.D. *Homeopathy: Beyond Flat Earth Medicine.* San Diego: Timing Publications, 1995.

Eskinazi, D. "Homeopathy Re-revisited: Is Homeopathy Compatible with Biomedical Observations?" *Archives of Internal Medicine* 159 (September 1999).

Golden, I. "Homeopathic Disease Prevention." *Homeopathy Online* (December 2000). (Web site: www.lyghtforce.com).

Hahnemann, S. *Organon of the Medical Art.* W. B. O'Reilly, Ph.D., ed. Palo Alto, Calif.: Birdcage Press, 2001.

Hoover, T. A. "Homeopathic Prophylaxis: Fact or Fiction." *Journal of the American Institute of Homeopathy* (Autumn 2001).

Hoover, T. A. "Smallpox: A Homeopathic Perspective." *Homeopathy Today* (January 2003).

Hyde, R. C. "Homeopathic Prophylaxis? Tantalizing Question, Surprising Answer." *Homeopathy Today* (December 2001).

"Immunization Advice from the Experts: Five Homeopaths Answer Your Most Frequently Asked Questions." *Homeopathy Today* (May–June 2004).

Johnson, A. G. "Surgery as Placebo." *Lancet* 344, no. 8930 (1994).

Jonas, W. B. "Do Homeopathic Nosodes Protect Against Infection? An Experimental Test." *Alternative Therapies in Health and Medicine* 5, no. 5 (September 1999).

Kent, J. T. *Repertory of the Homeopathic Materia Medica*. Lancaster, England: Examiner Printing House, 1897.

Kleijnen, J., et al. "Clinical Trials of Homoeopathy." *British Medical Journal* 302 (February 9, 1991).

Lansky, A. *Impossible Cure: The Promise of Homeopathy*. Portola Valley, Calif.: R. L. Ranch, 2003.

Linde, K., et al. "Are the Clinical Effects of Homeopathy Placebo Effects? A Meta-analysis of Placebo-Controlled Trials." *Lancet* 350, no. 9081 (September 20, 1997).

Little, D. "The Origin of Homoeo-Prophylaxis." (Web site: www.simillimum.com /thelittlelibrary/homoeopathicphilosophy/prophylaxis.html).

Merrell, W. C., and Shalts, E. "Homeopathy." *Medical Clinics of North America* 86, no. 1 (2002).

Morrison, R. *Desktop Companion to Physical Pathology*. Grass Valley, Calif.: Hahnemann Clinic, 1998.

Morrison, R. "Research . . . and Rediscovery of a Cherished Remedy." *Homeopathy Today* (November 2002).

Panos, M., M.D., and Heimlich, J. *Homeopathic Medicine at Home*. Los Angeles: Tarcher, 1980.

Reichenberg-Ullman, J., N.D., M.S.W., and Ullman, R., N.D. *Rage-Free Kids: Homeopathic Medicine for Defiant, Aggressive, and Violent Children*. New York: Prima Lifestyles, 1999.

Reichenberg-Ullman, J., N.D., M.S.W., and Ullman, R., N.D. *Ritalin-Free Kids: Safe and Effective Homeopathic Medicine for ADHD and Other Behavioral and Learning Problems*. New York: Three Rivers Press, 2000.

Shalts, E. "The Heat Is On." *Homeopathy Today* (July/August 2001).

Shalts, E. "Two Different 'Faces' of Terror: Belle Harbor Plane Crash." *Homeopathy Today* (September 2002).

Shalts, E. "Homeopathy Changes Our Children's Lives." *Homeopathy Today* (October 2002).

Shalts, E. *"Homeopathy" in Integrative Medicine*. B. Kligler and R. A. Lee, eds. New York: McGraw-Hill Professional, 2004.

Vithoulkas, G. *The Science of Homeopathy*. New York: Grove Atlantic, 1980.

Vithoulkas, G. *Homeopathy: Medicine of the New Man*. New York: Fireside, 1985.

Vithoulkas, G. *A New Model for Health and Disease*. Berkeley, Calif.: North Atlantic Books, 1992.

Winston, J. *The Faces of Homeopathy*. Tawa, New Zealand: Great Auk Publishing, 1999.

Winston, J. "From the Editor: The Medicalization of Life." *Homeopathy Today* (November 2002).

Yasgur, J. *Yasgur's Homeopathic Dictionary and Holistic Health Reference*. Greenville, Penn.: Vann Hoy, 1998.

Resources

General Information

Edward Shalts M.D., D.Ht.
Museum West Medical
123 West 79th Street, Suite PH4
New York, New York 10024
(212) 362-1884
www.homeopathynewyork.com

Dr. Shalts' AIH Remedy Kit for Parents is available through this Web site:
www.1-800homeopathy.com.

American Institute of Homeopathy (AIH)
801 North Fairfax Street, Suite 306
Alexandria, Virginia 22314-1757
(888) 445-9988
www.homeopathyusa.org

Professional and Public Organizations

The following organizations are provided to help you find a homeopath and any additional information you may desire.

American Board of Homeotherapeutics (ABHt)
1913 Gladstone Drive
Wheaton, Illinois 60187
(630) 668-5595
www.homeopathyusa.org

California Homeopathic Medical Society (CHMS)
169 East El Roblar Drive
Ojai, California 93023
(805) 646-1495
www.homeopathywest.org

Council for Homeopathic Certification (CHC)
P.M.B. 187
17051 Southeast 272nd Street, Suite 43
Covington, Washington 98042
(866) 242-3399 (toll free)
www.homeopathicdirectory.com

Council on Homeopathic Education (CHE)
91 Cornell Street
Newton, Massachusetts 02462-1320
(617) 244-8780
www.chedu.org

Florida Homeopathic Medical Society
668 Lake Villas Drive
Altamonte Springs, Florida 32701
(407) 628-9708
prswan@aol.com

Homeopathic Medical Society
of the State of New York (HMSSNY)
6250 Route 9
Rhinebeck, New York 12572
(845) 876-6323
homeopathicmd@earthlink.net

Homeopathic Nurses Association (HNA)
8403 Tahona Drive
Silver Spring, Maryland 20903
(301) 445-0611
www.homeopathicnurses.org

Homœopathic Pharmacopœia Convention
of the United States (HPCUS)
P.O. Box 2221
Southeastern, Pennsylvania 19399-2221
(610) 783-0987
www.HPCUS.com

Illinois Homeopathic Medical Association
400 East 22nd Street, Suite F
Lombard, Illinois 60148
(630) 792-9311

National Center for Homeopathy (NCH)
801 North Fairfax Street, Suite 306
Alexandria, Virginia 22314
(703) 548-7790
www.homeopathic.org

NCH publishes a magazine called *Homeopathy Today*. It is open to the general public for membership, and anyone can attend its annual conferences. Additionally, NCH sponsors Affiliated Study Groups for anyone who wants to learn more about using homeopathy for home use.

National Board of Homeopathic Examiners (NBHE)
6536 Stadium Drive, Suite L
Zephyrhills, Florida 33542
(813) 782-2690
www.nbhe.org

Ohio State Homeopathic Medical Society (OSHMS)
5779 Wooster Pike
Medina, Ohio 44256
(330) 784-4493

Texas Society of Homeopathy
4200 Westheimer, Suite 100
Houston, Texas 77027
(713) 621-3184
www.txsoho.com

Information Services and Booksellers

Homeopathic Educational Services
2124 Kittredge Street, Suite N
Berkeley, California 94704
(800) 359-9051
www.homeopathic.com

HomeopathyWest
1442A Walnut Street, #138
Berkeley, California 94709
(877) 850-5078
www.HomeopathyWest.com

Kent Homeopathic Associates
710 Mission Avenue
San Rafael, CA 94901

WholeHealthNow
#611-1733 H Street, Suite 330
Blaine, Washington 98230
(866) 599-5950
www.wholehealthnow.com

Minimum Price Homeopathic Books
250 H Street
P.M.B. 2187
Blaine, Washington 98230
(800) 663-8272 (orders only)
www.minimum.com

Educational Organizations and Programs

Colorado Institute for Classical Homeopathy
P.O. Box 20340
Boulder, Colorado 80308-3340
(303) 440-3717
www.homeopathyschool.org

Desert Institute School of Classical Homeopathy
2001 West Camelback Road, #150
Phoenix, Arizona, 85015
(602) 347-7950
www.weteachhomeopathy.com

Florida Academy of Classical Homeopathy
320 West Minnesota Avenue
Deland, Florida 32720-3350
(386) 736-8685
www.floridahomeopathy.org

The Institute of Natural Health Sciences Council on Homeopathic Education
(CHE) Professional Accreditation
20270 Middlebelt Road, Suite 4
Livonia, Michigan 48152
(248) 473-8522
www.naturalhealthsciences.org

Nashville School of Homeopathy
1929 21st Avenue South
Nashville, Tennessee 37212
(615) 477-2019
www.homeopathytennessee.com

New England School of Homeopathy (NESH)
356 Middle Street
Amherst, Massachusetts 01002
(413) 256-5949
www.nesh.com

Northwestern Academy of Homeopathy
5201 Eden Avenue, Suite 245
Minneapolis, Minnesota 55436
(612) 794-6445
www.homeopathicschool.org

Southwest College of Naturopathic Medicine
2140 East Broadway Road
Tempe, Arizona 85282
(480) 858-9100
www.scnm.edu

The Texas Institute for Homeopathy
1406 Brookstone
San Antonio, Texas 78248-1425
(210) 492-3162
www.texashomeopathy.com

Suppliers of Homeopathic Remedies

Annandale Apothecary and Health Center
3299 Woodburn Road, Suite 120
Annandale, Virginia 22003
(703) 698-7411
pfhughes1@verizon.net

Arrowroot Standard Direct
83 East Lancaster Avenue
Paoli, Pennsylvania 19301
(800) 234-8879
www.arrowroot.com

The Apothecary
5415 West Cedar Lane
Bethesda, Maryland 20814
(800) 869-9159
www.The-Apothecary.com

C. O. Bigelow Chemists
414 Avenue of the Americas
New York, New York 10011
(212) 473-7324
www.bigelowchemists.com

Boericke & Tafel, a division of Nature's Way Products
1375 North Mountain Springs Parkway
Springville, Utah 84663
(800) 962-8873
www.naturesway.com

Boiron
6 Campus Boulevard
Newtown Square, Pennsylvania 19073
(800) 264-7661 (store location service)
www.boiron.com

Budget Pharmacy
3001 Northwest 7th Street
Miami, Florida 33125
(800) 221-9772
budgetrx@aol.com

Dolisos America
3014 Rigel Avenue
Las Vegas, Nevada 89102
(800) 365-4767
www.dolisosamerica.com

Hahnemann Laboratories Inc.
1940 4th Street
San Rafael, California 94901
(888) 427-6422 (toll free)
www.hahnemannlabs.com

Homeopathy Works
33 Fairfax Street
Berkeley Springs, West Virginia 25411
(800) 336-1695
www.homeopathyworks.com

Mediral International Inc.
10550 East 54th Avenue, Unit E
Denver, Colorado 80239-2131
(877) 633-4725 (toll free)
www.mediral.com

Merz Apothecary
4716 North Lincoln Avenue
Chicago, Illinois 60625
(800) 252-0275
www.smallflower.com

Natural Health Supply (NHS) Labs
6410 Avenida Christina
Santa Fe, New Mexico 87507
(888) 689-1608
www.a2zhomeopathy.com

1-800-HOMEOPATHY
P.O. Box 8080
Richford, Vermont 05476
(800) 466-3672
www.1800homeopathy.com

Santa Monica Homeopathic Pharmacy
629 Broadway
Santa Monica, California 90401
(310) 395-1131
www.smhomeopathic.com

Standard Homeopathic Company
210 West 131st Street
P.O. Box 61067
Los Angeles, California 90061
(800) 624-9659
www.hylands.com

Washington Homeopathic Products Inc.
4914 Del Ray Avenue
Bethesda, Maryland 20814
(800) 336-1695
www.homeopathyworks.com

Weise Pharmacy, Homeopathic and Natural Medicines
4343 Colonial Avenue
Jacksonville, Florida 32210
(800) 554-6670
www.weiserx.com

About the Author

Edward Shalts, M.D., D.Ht., is trustee of the American Institute of Homeopathy and vice president of the National Center for Homeopathy. Born and raised in Russia, he graduated from medical school in Moscow. He practiced family medicine and homeopathy there until 1988, when he immigrated to the United States. For four years following his arrival, Dr. Shalts worked as a postdoctoral research scientist at Columbia University. He then completed psychiatric residency training at the Beth Israel Medical Center in New York City, where he served as chief resident. Afterward, he practiced homeopathy, conducted research, and taught for four years at the Continuum Center for Health and Healing, one of the largest centers of complementary and alternative medicine in the world, which is affiliated with the Beth Israel Medical Center. Currently, Dr. Shalts remains on the center's faculty and also has a private practice in New York City. He is a diplomate both of the American Board of Homeotherapeutics and of the American Board of Psychiatry and Neurology and is a founding diplomate of the American Board of Holistic Medicine. The father of two daughters, Dora and Polina, he lives in New Jersey with his wife, Natasha.

Index